GETTING PREGNANT
What Couples Need to
Know Right Now

GETTING PREGNANT

What Couples Need to Know Right Now

NIELS H. LAUERSEN, M.D., Ph.D.

AND

COLETTE BOUCHEZ

FAWCETT COLUMBINE NEW YORK

A Fawcett Columbine Book
Published by Ballantine Books

Library of Congress Catalog Card Number: 91-90651
ISBN: 0-449-90667-1

Cover design by Kristine V. Mills
Cover photo: Elyse Lewin/The Image Bank

Manufactured in the United States of America

First Ballantine Books Edition: July 1992

20 19 18 17 16 15 14 13

This book is not intended as a substitute for medical advice of physicians. The reader should regularly consult a physician in matters relating to his or her health, particularly with respect to any symptoms that may require diagnosis or medical attention.

Acknowledgments

Through the course of writing this book, many friends, colleagues and patients have blessed us with their support, enthusiasm, insights, and knowledge. We thank each of them for every contribution, and for caring about this book.

In particular, we would like to thank the following experts in the field of reproductive medicine who, through their own achievements and research, helped us to better understand the subject of fertility: Richard Amelar, M.D.; Ricardo Asch, M.D.; Professor Ian Craft; Gary D. Hodgen, Ph.D.; Georgeanna Seegar Jones, M.D.; Howard W. Jones, M.D.; Jonathan Scher, M.D.; John Stangel, M.D.; Zev Rosenwaks, M.D.

A special acknowledgment to Hugh K. Barber, M.D., Director of Obstetrics and Gynecology at Lenox Hill Hospital, for his insights, and for helping to establish new and higher standards of health care for women.

A very special thank you to J. Victor Reyniak, M.D., chief of Reproductive Endocrinology, Mt. Sinai Medical Center, New York, for unselfishly sharing his knowledge and his time.

Our gratitude also goes to Joyce Zeitz and the American Fertility Society; Sharon Danna and 9 To 5—the National Organization of Working Women; RESOLVE; and Erik Jansson and the National Network to Prevent Birth Defects, for sharing their research and their insights.

We would also like to thank the entire staff of the New York Medical Service for Reproductive Medicine for their valuable insights and contributions, particularly Majid Fateh, M.D.; Louise Weidel, Ph.D.; Magda Binion, M.D.; and Neil Ratner, M.D.

A very sincere and special thank you goes to Dr. Yanni Antonopolous, whose wisdom, knowledge, friendship, and support we deeply appreciate.

We would also like to thank Adrian Rothenberg for her photographic contributions and Ronnie Verebay for her administrative assistance.

Our respect and appreciation go to our legal advisors, Harvey Sindel and Stuart Altman.

Our thanks also go to the staff of Rawson Associates and the Macmillan Publishing Company, most especially Carol Cook.

We would also like to thank Grace Shaw for her valuable insights and comments on the manuscript.

Our most sincere appreciation goes to Barry Lippman, president of the Macmillan Publishing Company, for believing in this project.

Finally, our deepest gratitude goes to our editor and publisher Eleanor Rawson, whose insights, wisdom, encouragement, and support guided this book to completion. Thank you for always being there.

NIELS H. LAUERSEN, M.D., PH.D.
COLETTE BOUCHEZ

CONTENTS

vii

· II ·

THE FASTEST, EASIEST WAYS TO A SAFE NATURAL CONCEPTION

◆ Can You Try Too Hard to Get Pregnant? ◆ Can Sweat
Make You More Fertile? ◆ Getting Pregnant After Thirty-
five ◆ One Dozen Super New and Time-tested Ways to
Encourage Natural Conception at Any Age!

· III ·

IF YOU DON'T GET PREGNANT RIGHT AWAY . . . HOW SCIENCE CAN HELP YOU CONCEIVE!

◆ IV ◆

YOUR PERSONAL PREGNANCY PLANNER

INTRODUCTION: THE REALLY GOOD NEWS ABOUT GETTING PREGNANT

When I was in medical school in the 1960s, young men and women were far more concerned with avoiding pregnancy than with getting pregnant. The birth control pill, not prenatal vitamins, was the prescription of the decade. Happily, getting pregnant is no longer something most couples want to avoid, but a joyous, life-expanding experience to be celebrated and cherished. Along with these new changes in attitude, came some equally important scientific advancements that made it faster and easier for all couples to achieve their parenting goals:

- New information about both male and female biologies have given us ways to encourage not only faster, but healthier conceptions, with fewer chances for miscarriage and birth defects.
- New information on the causes of infertility show how men and women can protect their fertility and their sex lives while they *safely* postpone childbearing.
- Advances made in the treatment of infertility—medications, micro-surgery, and laboratory assistance—are not only helping infertile couples to get pregnant, but are helping all couples over thirty-five to have safer, healthier pregnancies.

In fact, thanks to what has been learned in just the past three years alone, almost every couple who wants to have a baby, can have one!

WHY I WROTE THIS BOOK

Although the field of reproductive medicine is currently exploding with new advances, my deep commitment to fertility research goes back more than twenty years. As a member of several key scientific teams I have devoted thousands of hours to reproductive research, and my work has taken me around the world more than three times—to the capitals of Europe, where the first test tube babies were conceived, to the Soviet Union, to South America, to the Far East—anywhere I could learn the latest information on the reproductive system. In the past several years I joined forces with a team of dedicated physicians and researchers to create a clinic to utilize much of what has been learned. As a result, I have been able to see first hand the exciting, almost miraculous ways that much of the new reproductive technology can change people's lives.

- ◆ Couples who were thought to be hopelessly infertile are now able to conceive and deliver not one, but two and three perfect children.
- ◆ Those who previously miscarried up to fifteen times are now giving birth to healthy, full-term babies.

Time and again my colleagues and I witnessed a dramatic rise in the number of our patients over age thirty-five able to have all natural conceptions and healthy pregnancies thanks to a few simple dietary and lifestyle changes. Equally significant is the increase in the number of women under age thirty who are able to sail through their pregnancies without a single problem.

As I traveled in this country, however, giving lectures and making television appearances, I began to see that too many couples were not taking advantage of all the possibilities. Some of the new research had made its way to the general public, but many couples remained in the dark about their reproductive health. Much important information about getting pregnant remained within the confines of the medical establishment.

Thus, I conceived the idea for this book—a source for the newest and most important fertility information—data that I have seen make a difference in my patients' lives. It is my hope that it will make a difference in your life as well, whenever in your childbearing years you decide to get pregnant.

PART ONE: HOW THE NEW DISCOVERIES CAN HELP YOU

Whether you are planning to have a baby in the very near future, or even if you haven't decided when motherhood will be right for you, by knowing the factors that could affect your childbearing potential, you can take the necessary steps to protect your reproductive options and ensure that your body remains ready for pregnancy throughout your childbearing years. Part One of this book was developed to help you do just that.

It begins by exploring the very latest information on how your reproductive system functions and what biological factors can cause it to malfunction. It also explains how you can use your family history to help *predict* fertility problems, and it discusses the preventative treatments you need right now. It also shows how the ways that you and your partner live, work, and play may be affecting your reproductive health, and it tells what you both can do, starting today, to make the most of your most fertile years. More of what you will discover in Part One includes:

- The important new link between great sex and super fertility
- How to tell if your job is harming your reproductive health
- The influence of the alcohol, caffeine, medication, and recreational drugs you are consuming today upon your ability to conceive tomorrow
- The kinds of birth control to safely postpone a pregnancy without harming your fertility

In addition, you will learn about a brand-new OB-GYN exam that offers you increased protection not only against infertility, but other important health concerns as well. You will discover what your doctor should be doing today to ensure your good health and protect your childbearing options tomorrow. Finally, you will learn the whole truth about male fertility, along with vital *new* ways your partner can protect his virility *and* his potency, while decreasing *your* risk of miscarriage and protecting your baby from birth defects.

PART TWO: GETTING PREGNANT RIGHT NOW—MORE GOOD NEWS!

If you are thinking about getting pregnant in the near future, and especially if you are actively trying to conceive right now, Part Two was written for you. It provides the latest information on everything in today's world capable of influencing your immediate ability to get pregnant. Some of what you will find in this section includes:

- Breakthrough treatments for preventing miscarriage—and what you can do *before* you conceive to reduce your risk
- The new link between dieting and conception—and how to find your ideal fertility weight
- How your fitness workouts can block a pregnancy—plus the exercises that can help you get pregnant faster
- How stress affects conception

- How to avoid major pregnancy complications
- How to get pregnant fast—plus five important things every woman over thirty-five *must* do before she tries to conceive
- The sexual practices and positions that encourage conception, and those that can block it—plus ways that lovemaking can influence the sex of your child!

In addition, you will find a new kind of nutritional guide with information on the foods and vitamins that can make you more fertile, help you avoid birth defects, and decrease your risk of miscarriage—along with a diet developed to help you get pregnant!

Finally, you'll learn about preconception counseling, the brand-new way couples are helping to ensure their pregnancy, plus twelve up-to-date ways to encourage a faster, easier conception. You'll even learn how making love on your birthday might help you get pregnant!

PART THREE: IF YOU DON'T GET PREGNANT RIGHT AWAY—WHAT TO DO

In Part Three you will find the newest and most important technological advances developed to help you have a baby even if you believe you are infertile. The data in Part Three will help you understand why you are having a problem getting pregnant, and it will also acquaint you with the multitude of opportunities for solving your problem. Some of what this section offers:

- How to tell if you can have a baby long before you try to conceive—plus how to turn any pregnancy odds in your favor
- Superovulation—one of the newest ways for every woman to increase her chance for conception
- The surprising truth about fertility drugs—and how they can help you have a *natural* conception
- The brand-new time-saving, money-saving fertility surgeries that require no hospitalization—and can help you get pregnant in record time!

Because we now know that male infertility is behind the conception difficulties of up to 40 percent of all couples who cannot conceive, this section will also help you discover the fastest, easiest ways your partner can overcome his fertility problems.

In addition, you'll learn the astonishing *new* ways that artificial insemination is helping millions of couples to get pregnant, and you'll find information on the breakthroughs that can increase the success of all laboratory-aided conceptions, including in vitro fertilization. Now, know—before you try—which method is right for you!

Finally, you'll learn about the GIFT procedure, the very newest reproductive technology, which can help you have a faster, easier, healthier conception, especially if you are over age thirty.

PART FOUR: YOUR PERSONAL PREGNANCY PLANNER

In Part Four of this book you'll find a Personal Pregnancy Planner, a six-month guide that takes you, step by step, through everything you need to do to have a perfect, healthy baby, whether you conceive naturally on your own or with laboratory assistance.

Whether showing you ways to protect your fertility from current dangers or helping you restore it from past dangers, the programs in this book were developed to help you and your partner have a faster, easier, healthier conception and pregnancy than was ever before possible. Not only can you be sure of your ability to get pregnant right now, but you can retain your reproductive options throughout your childbearing years.

The really good news about getting pregnant? *You* have the power! Good luck—and go for it!

I

◆

NEW DISCOVERIES ABOUT GETTING PREGNANT

What Affects Fertility

◆

· 1 ·

HOW YOUR BODY
WORKS

The Latest News

From the first moment you saw him smile, you knew he was the man for you. Well, perhaps it didn't happen quite that quickly. Maybe you dated each other for months or possibly even years before that mysterious and very wonderful feeling took over and you knew you were in love.

Regardless of when in your relationship it occurred, if you are like many women, finding that special someone may have elicited another, even more powerful feeling: the desire to have a baby. While childbearing was once the farthest thing from her mind, many an obstetrical patient has told me that from almost the instant she met her mate her *babylust* began.

For other women, however, things can work just the opposite: the desire for motherhood may come long before a potential partner appears. In fact, some patients confide to me that it was their unrelenting desire to *have* a baby that prompted their search for a soul-mate—or at least a suitable parenting partner!

While no one is really certain *what* causes a woman's baby alarm to ring, the recognition that it exists was one of the elements that led researchers to a key discovery about how and why you get pregnant. What was it they discovered? The vital role of reproductive hormones.

It was once believed that getting pregnant was strictly a physiological function of your reproductive organs, but today research shows that the same biochemicals that influence your desire to have a baby also play a key role in helping you achieve conception. In fact, without your reproductive hormones, you could *not get* pregnant!

3

THE NEW CONCEPTION CHEMISTRY:
HOW IT WORKS

From the moment puberty starts and throughout your childbearing years, your body and your brain work together in a unique biological partnership, to produce a series of chemicals called reproductive hormones.

Research shows that the activity of your reproductive hormones can affect everything from your mood to your desire for sex—even your appetite for certain foods. Some new studies also suggest that hormones are what cause a woman's *baby alarm* to ring, stimulating a natural *mothering* instinct, the feeling perceived as a desire to get pregnant.

The strength of this feeling and when (and how often) in your childbearing years it occurs are also thought to be influenced, at least in part, by hormonal activity.

Even more important, however, is the way hormones affect your ability to get pregnant. Although the total number of eggs your ovaries can produce is predetermined *before* you are born (in most women, about 400,000 follicles exist), we now know that for you to *get* pregnant these follicles must be able to develop and grow and then be released from your ovary into your fallopian tube. Ultimately they must be able to be fertilized, and finally, your embryo must implant into your uterus, and grow as well. While it is your reproductive *organs* that actually perform these vital tasks, the latest research shows that it is your reproductive *hormones* that provide the biochemical signals necessary to put these organs into motion.

THE HORMONES THAT HELP YOU GET
PREGNANT

All told, five reproductive hormones are necessary for conception. They send their signals to your various organs by rising and falling in a distinct and carefully timed pattern throughout the course of a single monthly menstrual cycle. The effects of all five are felt in your body, but three of these hormones are continually being manufactured and released into your bloodstream, by your brain. The first two are:

Follicle-stimulating hormone (FSH). Secreted by your pituitary gland (which is located at the base of your brain), it stimulates the follicles inside your ovaries to produce eggs.

Lutenizing hormone (LH). Also secreted by your pituitary gland, it signals to your egg when the time is right to leave your ovary and be ovulated into your fallopian tube so that fertilization can take place.

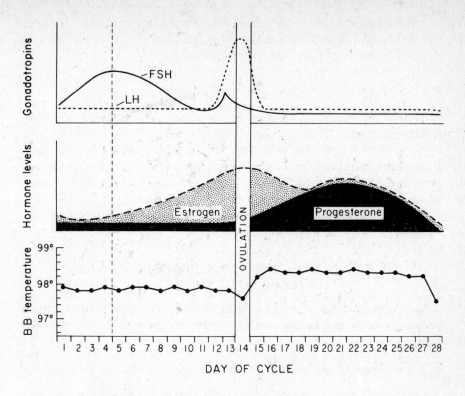

The Hormones That Help You Get Pregnant

In order for you to get pregnant, your body must maintain a fine biochemical balance among the four reproductive hormones: FSH (follicle stimulating hormone), LH (luteinizing hormone), estrogen, and progesterone. Hormone levels rise and fall in distinct patterns throughout each menstrual cycle, and changes in your body temperature reflect changes in the hormone balances. The ebb and flow of all these factors work together to create your fertility curve—the time of the month when you can conceive.

Collectively they are called gonadotropins. Although some FSH and LH remain in your body at all times, both are secreted in great amounts during the first half of your menstrual cycle, and levels of both drop sharply after ovulation. It was recently discovered that in order for this fluctuation to occur, another hormone must enter the fertility equation:

> *Gonadotropin-releasing hormone* (GnRH). This helps release the proper amounts of gonadotropins (FSH and LH) into your bloodstream. Secreted by your hypothalamus, a tiny gland located near your pituitary, GnRH functions as a kind of biochemical radar system that pulses through your body every 90 to 120 minutes,

twenty-four hours a day. It monitors your bloodstream for levels of FSH and LH and then at the proper time directs your pituitary to release more of each into your bloodstream.

BALANCING YOUR FERTILITY EQUATION

Getting pregnant also requires estrogen and progesterone, two more fertility hormones. They are manufactured in your ovaries (and elsewhere in your body) and also rise and fall in a precisely timed pattern throughout each menstrual cycle. Their purpose is to orchestrate various steps in the egg production and release process, which you'll read more about later in this chapter.

After you become pregnant it is estrogen and progesterone that help maintain your pregnancy and protect you from miscarriage.

GETTING READY TO GET PREGNANT: HOW YOUR BODY WORKS

Each month, at the start of every menstrual cycle, your body begins to prepare you for a new opportunity to get pregnant. This is a five-step process.

STEP 1: EGG PRODUCTION

Starting on the first day of your menstrual cycle (the day you start to bleed), your GnRH messengers sense that FSH is low. In turn your hypothalamus gland sends a signal to your pituitary to begin producing and releasing more of this hormone into your bloodstream. The purpose is to stimulate a new group of follicles inside your ovary to begin producing eggs.

STEP 2: GETTING YOUR UTERUS READY

As your eggs start to grow, the follicles release estrogen. In a natural anticipation of fertilization, these rising estrogen levels stimulate the tissue that lines the inside of your uterus (called the endometrium) to begin growing thicker. This helps to form a spongy nest into which your embryo (the fertilized egg) can easily implant and start to grow.

STEP 3: SELECTING THE EGG OF THE MONTH

Within a few days after the stimulation of your egg follicles, one of them begins to surpass the others in growth and maturity. Called the graafian follicle, it produces what is thought to be the strongest egg, the one you will eventually ovulate.

OVULATION AND FERTILIZATION

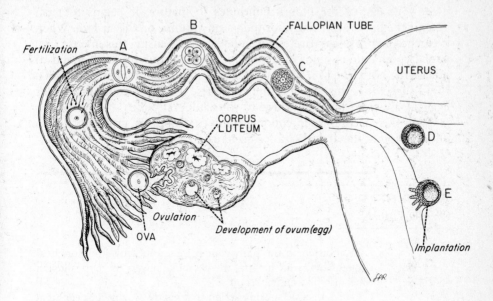

Getting Pregnant: How Your Body Works

At the start of each menstrual cycle, your hypothalamus gland (located in your brain) releases the hormone GnRH (gonadotropin releasing hormone). This signals your pituitary gland (also located in your brain) to release FSH (follicle stimulating hormone), which in turn stimulates the follicles inside your ovaries to begin producing eggs. As the eggs begin to grow, they release the hormone estrogen, which in turn encourages the lining of your uterus (the endometrium) to begin growing as well, in anticipation of receiving a fertilized egg.

After approximately twelve to fourteen days your egg is ripe and mature enough to be fertilized. A sharp rise in estrogen triggers your pituitary to release still another hormone, LH (luteinizing hormone), which signals your egg to pop from its shell and leave your ovary (ovulation). As it does, the fimbria, the fingerlike ends of your fallopian tube, reach down and catch it, and guide it inside.

The deserted shell your egg leaves behind (called the corpus luteum) begins producing the hormone progesterone, which helps to prepare your uterus further for implantation of a fertilized egg.

In the meantime, sperm, which have been deposited in your vagina, swim through your cervix, into your uterus, and down into both fallopian tubes, in anticipation of meeting your egg. Your cervical mucus aids in the transport. In order for a pregnancy to occur, however, sperm must make contact with your egg within twelve to twenty-four hours after ovulation. After this time your egg begins to disintegrate and pregnancy generally does not occur.

Sperm must get inside your egg during this same time frame. To help accomplish this, the head of each sperm (the acrosome) is filled with enzymes that are immediately released on contact with your egg. They help break down the outer coating and allow passage inside.

Once inside, the sperm membrane fuses with the membrane surrounding your egg, and an embryo is formed. Over the next three days, it divides several times. When it reaches the eight-cell stage, it is strong enough to begin traveling down the remainder of your fallopian tube and into your uterus—a journey that takes roughly five to seven days. When it arrives it will—hopefully—implant in your endometrium and begin to grow into a developing fetus.

STEP 4: OVULATION

As your egg of the month continues to mature, it begins to push against the top of your ovary, forming a tiny bubble on the surface. When it reaches its peak maturity, estrogen levels soar. Sensing this intense rise, your hypothalamus sends a second message to your pituitary gland to release the hormone LH, which also shoots into your bloodstream with a rapid surge. It is this fast and immediate rise in LH that stimulates your egg to leave your ovary and travel to your fallopian tube.

After this occurs, your endometrium continues to grow thicker in anticipation of the arrival of a fertilized egg.

WHAT HELPS OVULATION

In addition to the push your egg receives from the hormonal surge of LH, your fimbria, the petal-like fingers of your fallopian tube, also play an important role.

Using a gentle sucking action that gently coaxes your egg from its shell, your fimbria actually reach down and massage your ovary just prior to ovulation.

As your egg bursts through your ovary, the fimbria act like a fertility safety net, catching and gently guiding it inside your fallopian tube so that it can meet your partner's sperm and become fertilized.

STEP 5: GETTING PREGNANT

Once your egg is in your fallopian tube, it is ready to be fertilized, but it only remains fertile for about twelve to twenty-four hours, after which time it begins to disintegrate. In order for conception to occur, your partner's sperm must make contact with your egg within the twelve to twenty-four hours following ovulation. You'll learn later how you can ensure that this occurs.

HOW YOUR LIFE CYCLES CONTINUE TO FUNCTION

Whether or not you get pregnant, from the moment you ovulate, the follicle your egg leaves behind becomes a fully functioning endocrine gland. Called the corpus luteum, it continues producing estrogen (much the way your egg did) and begins producing progesterone, which helps

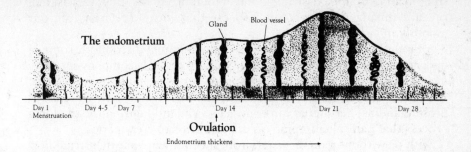

The endometrium

Gland   Blood vessel

| Day 1 | Day 4-5 | Day 7 | Day 14 | Day 21 | Day 28 |

Menstruation

Ovulation

Endometrium thickens

The menstrual cycle

The purpose of the menstrual cycle is to prepare the uterus, or womb, for possible pregnancy. During the cycle, the special endometrial tissue lining the inside of the uterus undergoes certain specific changes. It grows and thickens. Blood vessels and glands develop to provide a nourishing environment for the fertilized egg. The female sex hormones—estrogen and progesterone, secreted by the ovaries— are responsible for these changes. About the sixth day of the cycle, just after menstruation has ceased, the endometrium is no more than half a centimeter thick. Increasing levels of estrogen then induce the endometrium to grow so rapidly that, by the fourteenth day, it may be as much as *ten times* thicker than it was the week before.

The usual menstrual cycle is approximately four weeks long. Ovulation takes place in the middle of the cycle, on about day 14. The ovarian follicle breaks open to release the egg or ovum that has been developing in the ovary.

If the egg is fertilized, it completes its journey through the fallopian tube, passes into the uterine cavity, and attaches to the thickened endometrium on about day 22. Menstrual periods then cease until after delivery.

If the egg is *not* fertilized, estrogen and progesterone levels decline and the thickened endometrial tissue breaks down. Menstruation takes place as blood and endometrial tissue are discharged through the vagina. This completes one cycle; the reproductive organs are then ready for another cycle stimulated by the brain.

soften the lining of your uterus, and makes implantation easier, and therefore stronger. This can help you avoid miscarriage.

If you don't become pregnant (either by choice or for other reasons, discussed later in this book), your corpus luteum is preprogrammed to produce progesterone and estrogen for just fourteen days, after which time it begins to disintegrate. As it does, estrogen and progesterone levels drop sharply. Since without high levels of these hormones your spongy uterine lining cannot exist, it begins to disintegrate as well.

WHY YOU GET A MENSTRUAL PERIOD

To help cleanse your system of this now needless tissue, your body begins to produce a series of biochemicals called prostaglandins. They help stimulate powerful uterine contractions that pull the excess tissue from the walls of your uterus and expel it from your body. It is the combination of this tissue and the blood from the tiny vessels that rupture during the extracting process that forms the basis of your monthly menstrual flow.

Although this process should cause only minimal discomfort, some of my patients report pain ranging from mild to severe accompanying *every* menstrual period. Why does this happen? It was recently discovered that when, for various reasons, a woman produces extremely high levels of prostaglandins, her uterus can contract so violently during the shedding process that painful cramping occurs just prior to every period.

With or without pain, however, from the moment your menstrual flow begins, the entire hormonal network is reactivated, and your body begins to prepare for another twenty-eight-day cycle—and a new chance to get pregnant.

HOW YOUR PERSONAL BIOLOGY AFFECTS YOUR FERTILITY

In order for you to get pregnant at any time during your childbearing years, your body must maintain a finely balanced biochemical equilibrium. Unfortunately, current research shows this is not always possible. In fact, a woman's reproductive chemistry can be so fragile, that sometimes something as simple as a cold or flu or even not getting enough sleep can throw things out of sync. As a result you probably experience *short* spans of infertility far more often than you realize. This is one of the reasons you don't automatically get pregnant each time you have unprotected intercourse, even if relations take place at the time of ovulation.

More important, recent research has found that certain more serious personal biological factors can cause your fertility critical, long-lasting harm. If left untreated, some of these factors can render you permanently infertile.

YOU CAN PREVENT INFERTILITY!

The real importance of this increased understanding has not only been in isolating the biological factors that can harm your fertility (you'll learn what they are in the next chapter) but in recognizing that in many instances you, yourself, have the power to prevent harm from occurring.

Combined with the new methods your doctor has for identifying potential problems long before they exist, and a plethora of revolutionary, fast, and easy ways to treat those that do occur (all discussed in the next chapter), it's now possible to significantly reduce your risk of some of the major causes of infertility.

PERSONAL PREGNANCY POWER!

How can you begin to assume this new and exciting control over your reproductive fate? By becoming an active, aggressive, *educated* partner in your own fertility care. This is especially important if you are planning to preserve some of your childbearing options for the future. Why?

Very often the effects of reproductive damage are cumulative and *silent*: what is happening in your body today might not be evident for several more years. However, by remaining critically aware of what has the potential to harm you, you can catch most problems *before* significant damage has occurred. In this way you can have *total control* over your ability to get pregnant—both right now and in the future.

· 2 ·

SEVEN SUPER FERTILITY THREATS—AND HOW YOU CAN AVOID THEM

Not every physiological factor capable of affecting reproductive health will necessarily harm *your* fertility, of course, but recent research has shown that certain conditions do routinely affect a significant number of women. Although some of these factors are obvious (for example, the much publicized link between infertility and IUDs), some may not be so easy to see. Many of the patients who come to my fertility clinic are surprised, even shocked, to learn that the inability to conceive could be the result of conditions like endometriosis, fibroid tumors, or even simple infections that have gone undiagnosed and untreated for too long. For many, the signs of infertility are so subtle that problems are not even noticed until they decide to have a baby and find they cannot conceive.

How can you tell what aspects of your personal biology may be placing your fertility at risk? By listening to your body for the important signs and symptoms listed in this chapter and, when applicable, checking into your personal and family health history for factors that place you at high risk. Then, using this information, you and your doctor can work together to avoid or stop the most common and harmful threats to your fertility.

THREAT 1: ENDOMETRIOSIS

Endometriosis is a devastating menstrual-related disorder. It is thought to develop when blood and uterine lining, normally shed during your monthly menstrual cycle, are somehow thrown into a retrograde motion: instead of leaving your body, they are sprayed backward into your system.

Once inside, this material can land anywhere in your pelvic cavity, take root, and begin to grow, treating these organs as a sort of *substitute uterus*. Because this misplaced endometrial tissue is *nourished* each time your estrogen level climbs, as it does at the start of every menstrual cycle, it continues to grow month after month, continually being joined by new deposits left after every period.

ENDOMETRIOSIS: THE SYMPTOMS

- Severe menstrual cramps
- Ovulation pain (mittelschmerz)
- Pelvic pain that worsens before a period
- Dyspareunia (painful intercourse)
- Recurring bladder infections
- Painful pelvic cysts and tumors
- Lower back pain
- Nausea, vomiting, and dizziness during menstruation

Sometimes, however, endometriosis can have no symptoms at all.

HOW ENDOMETRIOSIS AFFECTS YOUR FERTILITY

I have devoted more than twenty years to researching and treating endometriosis.

In the thousands of cases I have seen, the most popular sites for endometrial deposits to grow are the ovaries, the fallopian tubes, and the uterus. These growths (or their resulting scar tissue) can cause obstruction so severe that, if treatment is not received, the organs themselves can cease to function. The most common fertility-related complications of endometriosis are:

- Blood-filled "chocolate" cysts (so named because of their chocolate-like texture and color), which form on the ovaries and restrict egg development and release

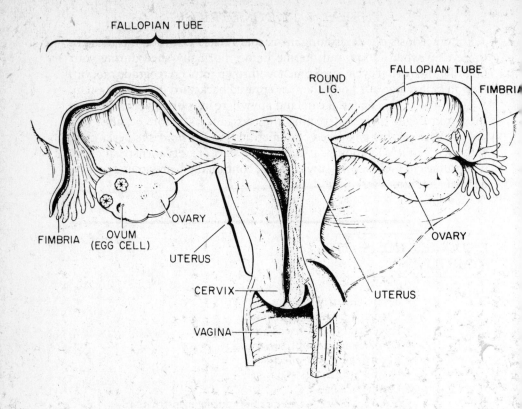

FALLOPIAN TUBE

ROUND LIG.

FALLOPIAN TUBE

FIMBRIA

FIMBRIA

OVUM (EGG CELL)

OVARY

UTERUS

CERVIX

VAGINA

OVARY

UTERUS

The Female Reproductive System

Enclosed in the bony structure of the pelvis are all of the organs necessary for reproduction:
◆ The vagina, the gateway to your reproductive tract.
◆ The cervix, or "mouth of the womb," the entrance to your uterus.
◆ The uterus, the layer of muscle that surrounds your endometrium, the cavity in which your baby will grow.
◆ The fallopian tubes, the two passageways leading from the ovaries to the uterus. They provide a route allowing sperm to get to your egg and a fertilized egg subsequently to reach your womb.
◆ The fimbria or tube ends. They help your egg to ovulate.
◆ The ovaries, which house your lifetime supply of egg follicles.

When any factor (such as disease, scar tissue, a cyst, or a tumor) blocks or restricts the function of any of these organs, or if a carelessly performed medical procedure (like an abortion or an IUD insertion) damages a portion of your system, your fertility can be placed at great risk.

- Damaged fimbria, whereby the fingerlike ends of the fallopian tubes stick together, blocking an ovulated egg from entering
- Intertubal blockage, which hampers egg transport or blocks sperm passage

When I first began to study endometriosis, I saw many patients whose condition had gone undiagnosed and untreated for so long that their lesions had turned into sticky masses of scar tissue that bound into a solid mass not only all their reproductive organs, but their bladder, bowels, and abdomen as well. For these women the only alternative was drastic surgery to save their lives.

HORMONES, ENDOMETRIOSIS, AND INFERTILITY

In addition to structural damage, I have also seen endometriosis affect fertility on a biochemical level, with problems that range from increased risk of miscarriage to complete inability to conceive. In 1980 Dr. Ter-

---

ENDOMETRIOSIS: ARE YOU AT RISK?

No one is really sure why some women get endometriosis and others do not. However, the following factors have been identified with increased risk:

- *Immune system deficiencies.* Although the backward bleeding of endometriosis is said to occur in every woman who menstruates, a healthy immune system is thought to be the line of defense that keeps the renegade tissue from taking root and growing. If a malfunction in your immune system occurs, this protection is suddenly lost, and you become a victim of endometriosis.
- *Stress.* I have observed that endometriosis proliferates or recurs in a woman's body faster and in greater quantity during times of extreme emotional stress, such as divorce, job loss, or the death of a spouse, parent, or other loved one.
- *Early menstrual periods.* If you experienced an early menstrual cycle (before age twelve) and your flow was exceptionally heavy at that time, you may be at higher risk for endometriosis.
- *Family history.* This disease can be hereditary. If your mother or another close female relative had endometriosis, studies at the Baylor College of Medicine in Texas reveal that you are seven times more likely to be afflicted by this problem than are women who have no family history of it.

---

rance Drake, head of reproductive endocrinology at the National Medical Center in Washington, D.C., conducted experiments that have helped us understand how and why this occurs. It was Dr. Drake who discovered that active endometrial lesions emit extraordinarily high levels of prostaglandin, the hormone-like chemical responsible for the severe menstrual cramps that often accompany this disease.

Much the way they normally cause your uterus to contract, an excess of prostaglandins can cause spasms in your fallopian tubes. If you should conceive, these spasms can move your fertilized egg to your uterus so quickly that it may not have the time to prepare adequately for a healthy implantation. The end result is often a miscarriage or premature labor. When combined with damage to the uterine lining, another effect of endometriosis, the risk of miscarriage becomes three times greater than normal.

Moreover, excessive prostaglandins in your body *before* you conceive can cause your internal environment to become so biochemically hostile that both sperm and egg are destroyed before fertilization can take place.

HOW TO PROTECT YOUR FERTILITY

As devastating as endometriosis can be, there *are* things you can do to protect yourself and your fertility even if you are at high risk. One of the best ways is through diet, which can help control the growth of any endometriosis that has already appeared and, in some cases, prevent it from occurring at all. In fact, I am continually amazed at how many of my patients are able to manage this problem—and in some cases even cure it completely—simply by eliminating certain foods from their diet.

What should you avoid eating if you are at high risk?

- ◆ High-fat dairy products:
  - ◆ cream cheese
  - ◆ high-fat yogurt
  - ◆ whole milk
  - ◆ cream
  - ◆ ice cream
  - ◆ cheese

The high fat content of these foods may stimulate an estrogen overload, which can accelerate the growth of endometrial tissue.

- ◆ Fresh fruit and fruit juices, including:
  - ◆ oranges
  - ◆ grapefruits
  - ◆ peaches
  - ◆ nectarines
  - ◆ melons

Nearly every fruit contains a natural substance called bioflavinoids, which has been linked to an excess of estrogen.

◆ Foods containing arachidonic acid (a saturated fat), an essential fatty acid, include:

- ◆ kidney
- ◆ liver
- ◆ red meat
- ◆ lard
- ◆ butter

Foods high in saturated fats can exacerbate inflammatory conditions like endometriosis.

WHAT SHOULD YOU EAT IF YOU HAVE ENDOMETRIOSIS?

A diet high in complex carbohydrates (grains, vegetables, and pasta), the skinless white meat of chicken and turkey, and broiled fish is recommended.

There is also evidence that foods containing GLA, another essential fatty acid may help counteract the effects of arachidonic acid. GLA can be found in cold-pressed sesame seed or walnut oil, and I recommend two tablespoons of either, once a day, if you have endometriosis.

Whenever possible eat natural foods that you cook yourself, rather than fast foods or the prepackaged variety, which are generally loaded with sodium, and can exacerbate some of your symptoms, especially abdominal cramping.

MORE WAYS TO PROTECT YOUR FERTILITY

Even if endometriosis does occur, it doesn't have to mean the end of your childbearing options. With early diagnosis and treatment, you can check it and help overturn most of its fertility-robbing consequences. In fact, with new medications and the advent of laser surgery, even the most severe damage can often be corrected, fertility and your partially or even fully restored.

What can help you?

- ◆ *Medications*. Since endometriosis needs estrogen to survive, medications that limit the production of this hormone allow your endometrial masses to shrivel and die. If treatment is received early enough, little or no scar tissue results. The three drugs currently used for this purpose are danazol (Danocrine), leuprolide acetate (Lupron), and Nafarelin. I have successfully prescribed these and have seen incredible results, often in a relatively short period of time.
- ◆ *Birth control pills*. Because they suppress your natural production of estrogen, I often prescribe birth control pills to prevent further development of mild cases of endometriosis. Although this is not a cure, I have seen it keep many women from succumbing to advanced stages of this disease.

◆ *Micro laser surgery.* Used to remove endometrial lesions and their resulting scar tissue, micro laser surgery, especially when teamed with danazol or leuprolide acetate (given three months prior to surgery and continued for three months afterward), can help most women experience a complete recovery and a total restoration of all reproductive functions. Studies are currently underway using Nafarelin for this same purpose.

PREGNANCY AND ENDOMETRIOSIS—A WARNING!

If endometriosis has not blocked your reproductive organs and you can conceive, your pregnancy may temporarily halt the spread of this problem. With no menstrual cycle for nine months, no new tissue can implant in your system. However, because estrogen levels soar during pregnancy, endometriosis that already exists may grow more rapidly, with serious consequences bearing on the outcome of the pregnancy itself. For this reason, *never accept pregnancy as a cure for endometriosis!*

For more information on this disease, see *The Endometriosis Answer Book* (New York: Rawson Associates, for hardcover; New York: Ballantine Books, for paperback).

THREAT 2: PELVIC INFLAMMATORY DISEASE

Although your reproductive functions are orchestrated by the hormonal activity that occurs in your brain, the conception of your child—and his or her subsequent growth and development—takes place within your body. The general area that houses your reproductive organs is your pelvis—a bony structure that contains your uterus, fallopian tubes, ovaries, and appendix, as well as part of your intestines, which are encased in a semiliquid membrane called the peritoneum. Should harmful bacteria, viruses, or other microorganisms make their way into your pelvic region, any number of serious fertility-robbing infections can result. Collectively called pelvic inflammatory disease (PID), they are specifically identified as follows:

◆ Endometritis: inflammation of the uterus
◆ Salpingitis: infection of the fallopian tube
◆ Oophoritis: ovarian infection
◆ Peritonitis: the most extreme form of PID, resulting in an infection of the entire pelvic cavity and the membrane surrounding the abdomen

Although technically almost anything that allows harmful micro-organisms to pass through your vagina and into your reproductive tract has the ability to bring about PID, there are several key factors that experts have observed (and I personally have found) to be most often responsible for these infections:

- Untreated sexually transmitted diseases (STDs) like gonorrhea and chlamydia (see Chapter Four)
- Use of an IUD
- A ruptured appendix
- An abortion performed under unsterile conditions

PID—THE SIGNS

The most obvious sign of PID is extreme pelvic pain, which can either build over a period of time or be sudden and severe.

Other warning signs can appear as well:

- Odorous vaginal discharge
- Painful urination
- Uterine bleeding
- Fever and chills
- Nausea and vomiting

Sometimes a woman with PID has no symptoms whatever or no more than a slight backache.

HOW PID AFFECTS YOUR FERTILITY

When diagnosed and treated early on, PID will usually not have a permanent effect on your fertility. However, as I often caution my patients, once these infections make their way inside your reproductive tract, there is always a chance for serious damage.

- If left untreated, the infections can cause your organs simply to deteriorate from disease, and their removal may be the only alternative. (Fortunately, the pain leading to this drastic stage is generally so severe that most infections are caught before surgery is necessary.)
- Even when cured, infections can leave scar tissue capable of blocking sperm and egg transport. Scarring can occur anywhere the diseased

tissue lived, but the most common sites are the inside lining of the fallopian tubes and the fimbria. If the scar tissue damage is severe, the fimbria can actually seal shut (a condition called clubbed tubes), in which case all chances for natural conception are lost.

PROTECTING YOUR FERTILITY FROM PID

The best way to protect your fertility from the ravages of PID, of course, is to be on the lookout for its earliest signs and symptoms, especially vaginal discharge and pelvic pain, and then seek treatment immediately. Sometimes your doctor can see or feel the presence of PID infections during your regular pelvic exam; at other times, a procedure called culdocentesis may be needed to lock in a diagnosis. Your doctor inserts a thin needle through your vagina into your abdominal cavity to aspirate fluid that is then tested for infection. In some extreme cases, I have found that a laparoscopy, a simple surgical technique that allows the doctor to view all the reproductive organs, is also helpful in confirming a diagnosis.

Once the diagnosis has been made, an antibiotic regimen taken for two to three weeks can help cure PID or check its spread. If need be, laser surgery can be performed later to help free the system of any scar tissue the infections may have left behind.

In addition, I have seen the following suggestions help protect many high-risk patients from contracting PID infection:

- ◆ Always use condoms when having sex with a high-risk partner (one who might have multiple partners or who displays any physical evidence of possible infection, especially abnormal penile discharge; see Chapter Four).
- ◆ Seek testing for STDs if you have had sex with someone you don't know well.
- ◆ Remain aware of the symptoms of all STDs (described in Chapter Four), and get tested at the first sign of infection.
- ◆ Recognize your high-risk factors: PID occurs more frequently if you are under age twenty-five, you have had a sexually transmitted disease and/or PID in the past, or you use an IUD (explained later in this chapter).

IF YOU HAVE HAD PID IN THE PAST ...

Don't panic now. As long as you received treatment, chances are your reproductive system did not suffer fertility-related traumas. However, I must caution you that because PID can leave behind an abundance of scar tissue, which can affect your ability to conceive, it may be a good idea to have your fertility checked *right now* even if you are not planning a pregnancy. Your doctor can do this with a simple procedure called a hysterosalpingogram, a special x-ray of your uterus and fallopian tubes, described in Chapter Fifteen.

If scar tissue is found, laser surgery can usually remove all traces and restore your fertility to optimum potential.

THREAT 3: FIBROID TUMORS

I don't think I have ever seen a patient who does not freeze with fear the moment her doctor uses the word *tumor*. As frightening as it sounds, however, I am always pleased to tell my patients that the majority of gynecological tumors are simple, *benign,* noncancerous growths that cause few, if any, life-threatening complications. This is especially true of fibroid tumors, the growth most often associated with fertility problems.

Composed of a solid mass of fibrous and muscular tissue, fibroids generally grow in and around the uterus, and therein lies their link to fertility. Ranging in size from a tiny seedling no bigger than a pea to melon-sized growths, fibroids are found both individually and in clusters (one patient of mine had thirty-two growing at the same time). Primarily, they interfere with conception by causing blockages in the reproductive tract.

WHERE, WHY, AND HOW FIBROID TUMORS GROW

The composition of all fibroid tumors is basically the same, and they all begin growing within the half-inch wall that surrounds your uterus. Based on the direction in which they grow, they are categorized into three types:

- *Intramural fibroid:* The most common type of fibroid, these remain within the wall of the uterus and are usually asymptomatic.
- *Subserous fibroid.* Rooted in the outer portion of the uterine wall, they push outward into the abdominal cavity and can sometimes form a stem at their base (called a pediculated fibroid). If that stem should twist (a common occurrence), it can result in pelvic pain that can be extremely severe. These fibroids can also cause pressure on the bladder, with pain prior to urination.
- *Submucous fibroid.* Pushing inward, these fibroids sometimes grow so large that they burst through the uterine lining and inflate the entire uterus. During the menstrual cycle, uterine contractions often attempt to push them out. This can cause severe pain and exceptionally heavy bleeding. If these growths also develop a "stem," they can dangle down into the cervix and cause pain during intercourse as well.

WHERE DO FIBROIDS COME FROM?

Studies show that 20 percent of all women between the ages of twenty and thirty-five and up to 30 percent of women over the age of thirty are the most susceptible to fibroids. I have rarely seen them in patients younger than twenty-five. Most often they begin growing when a woman is in her late twenties and early thirties and then continue throughout the childbearing years.

Because, as studies show, it is often high levels of estrogen that spark the growth of fibroid tumors, they can grow especially fast during pregnancy or if a woman is very overweight (see Chapter Nine). For this same reason, I have often seen them diminish and even disappear once a woman finishes menopause and estrogen levels drop dramatically. I have rarely seen a woman develop fibroids *after* menopause has been completed.

In addition to estrogen, these other factors can also make you more susceptible to fibroids:

- *Heredity*. There is strong evidence that fibroid tumors may run in families. If your mother or a close female relative had these growths, you may be at higher risk.
- *Predisposition*. Some women may be born with the fibroid seedlings already implanted. When they reach adulthood, some biochemical event sparks an excess of estrogen, which in turn exacerbates fibroid growth. This is why small tumors often grow like wildfire during pregnancy, when estrogen levels are constant and high.

HOW FIBROIDS AFFECT YOUR FERTILITY

Although I have seen a few patients who were not able to conceive due to excessively large intramural fibroids, the submucous tumors seem to cause the most fertility-related problems by far. When left to grow large enough, submucous fibroids can cause problems by:

- Interfering with the development of your endometrium, causing implantation problems and increasing your risk of miscarriage.
- Blocking your fallopian tube, keeping your fertilized egg from being transported to your uterus. When this happens, the embryo can sometimes start to grow inside your tube, resulting in an ectopic (out-of-womb) pregnancy. This is always fatal for your baby and potentially life threating for you. (See "Threat 7: Ectopic Pregnancy.")
- Altering the position of your cervix and by so doing keep your partner's sperm from passing into your uterus. This can prevent fertilization from taking place.

◆ Distorting the shape of your uterus, making implantation impossible or difficult; if conception occurs, this can increase your risk of miscarriage.

In addition, because the high levels of estrogen associated with pregnancy can make even the tiniest fibroid seedlings grow extremely large, if you do conceive when fibroids are present, studies indicate you may be at a somewhat higher risk for premature labor and/or miscarriage.

HOW YOU CAN PROTECT YOUR FERTILITY

The best way to protect your fertility against the damage of fibroid tumors is early diagnosis and treatment—if possible, long before you plan to conceive. By removing fibroids prior to conception, you can be sure that your uterus is clear for a healthy implantation.

I have found that one of the simplest treatments for fibroids is medication that decreases estrogen levels and creates a kind of *temporary menopause.* This can encourage tumors to shrink and disintegrate, much the way they often do when you undergo menopause naturally. These medications include danozol and leuprolide acetate (the same drugs used to treat endometriosis) and a promising new drug called simply LHRH, a synthetic version of several natural hormones that suppress estrogen levels by decreasing the activity of the pituitary gland. For most of my patients these medications have posed no significant side effects or problems. However, in a few patients I have observed certain drawbacks, primarily the onset of symptoms typical of menopause, such as hot flashes and a dry vagina, as well as temporary infertility. In addition, in some patients, fibroids resume growing as soon as the drugs are withdrawn.

CAN FIBROIDS DISAPPEAR ON THEIR OWN?

Sometimes—most often as a result of spontaneous changes in biochemistry. For this reason I sometimes prefer a wait-and-see attitude, so long as the fibroids are not interfering with conception. If your doctor offers you this alternative, be certain *not* to use birth control pills during this time. The estrogen they contain can spark the growth of your tumors or at least discourage their disintegration.

Because danazol can increase cholesterol levels, I believe it should not be used for more than six consecutive months, and blood cholesterol levels should be checked every few weeks during the time it is used.

THE FIBROID SURGERY THAT PRESERVES YOUR FERTILITY

Another option for treating fibroids is a myomectomy, a special type of surgery that removes only the tumors, leaving the rest of your reproductive organs intact. This is important to note, since many doctors still insist that a hysterectomy is the surgical treatment of choice for fibroid tumors.

If your doctor does suggest a hysterectomy for fibroids, I urge you to resist. This procedure will completely destroy your fertility, and every day evidence continues to mount that a hysterectomy for fibroid tumors is unnecessary for the majority of women in their reproductive years.

Conversely, a myomectomy, which removes your fibroids but leaves *all* your other reproductive organs intact, restores your fertility and will help you avoid the other catastrophic physical and emotional complications that directly follow a hysterectomy and can continue for life. You should consider a myomectomy if your fibroid tumors are causing you extreme pain or excessive bleeding or are clearly blocking your ability to conceive. For more information on myomectomy, see the chapter on fertility surgery in this book.

THREAT 4: OVARIAN CYSTS

If you have ever felt a sharp, nagging pain near your ovary, especially during ovulation or right before your period, you may already have experienced an ovarian cyst. Although for most women ovarian cysts come and go with only a temporary restriction of egg production or release, for others the condition can be more serious and present a more severe threat to fertility.

Different from a tumor in both structure and content, a cyst is a soft, fluid-filled sac that can appear in two different forms:

- *Functional cysts,* which are always benign and usually disappear on their own
- *Adenomas,* solid, long-lasting, potentially cancerous cysts that almost always have to be removed

Because at the onset it can be hard to distinguish between functional cysts and potentially malignant solid cysts, no ovarian growth should be dismissed or ignored. If I discover that a patient has an ovarian cyst, I make certain to examine her again after her next menstrual cycle—and possibly again the following month—to ensure that the growth is indeed disintegrating. In order to make an accurate diagnosis, sometimes a pelvic sonogram is also used, as well as a magnetic resonance image scanner (MRI), computerized tomographic (CT) scan, or even a laparoscopy. (These methods of internal visualization are explained in Chapter Seven.)

HOW CYSTS AFFECT YOUR FERTILITY

Regardless of the type of cyst, your fertility can be affected in a number of ways:

- If your ovary is covered by the cyst and is unable to function, your eggs can fail to develop. In addition, ovulation timing and function is disrupted and uterine preparation can be halted.
- If your cyst grows large enough, it can block your egg from leaving your ovary. This stops ovulation completely, and conception becomes impossible.
- If it turns out that your cysts are malignant (contain cancer cells), removal of part or all of your ovary may be indicated. Although you can conceive with as little as one quarter of one ovary, whenever a reproductive organ is removed, your fertility is compromised.

OVARIAN CYSTS: THE SYMPTOMS

How do you know you have an ovarian cyst and not just a stomach flu? Look for these symptoms to recur each month, in a cycle that worsens when you ovulate and right before your menstrual bleeding begins:

- Pain localized on one side of your abdomen
- Pain during ovulation
- Menstrual irregularities
- PMS
- Fever during ovulation or just prior to menstruation

Unfortunately, however, sometimes there are no symptoms.

PROTECTING YOUR FERTILITY: EARLY TREATMENT

In most cases I have found ovarian cysts to be temporary, disappearing on their own within two or three menstrual cycles. If they do affect fertility, it is usually only for a short time, and problems are normally resolved as soon as the cyst disappears.

To help promote the demise of cysts, I often prescribe birth control pills with a steady hormone level. Unlike the triphasic pills, which supply varying levels of hormones throughout the month and have been linked to the formation of ovarian cysts, pills that provide a constant level of hormones can encourage disintegration. When I come across a patient who, for one reason or another, does not respond to birth control pills, or when other health factors preclude their use, danazol has been successfully substituted.

If a cyst fails to disappear after two or three months, however, and especially if it does not respond to treatment, it may be one of three other types of ovarian growths, all having potentially serious fertility and health-related consequences:

- *Serous cystadenoma.* These are also known as the 50-50 cyst because they are malignant about 50 percent of the time and because they occur in both ovaries 50 percent of the time. They range from small to large and can cause various levels of discomfort.
- *Mucinous cystadenoma.* Filled with a thick fluid, these growths account for 10 to 15 percent of all malignant cysts; they are usually found on only one ovary. They can grow very rapidly and often become extremely large rather quickly. This can cause acute pain and discomfort.
- *Dermoid cysts.* Representing about 10 to 20 percent of all potentially malignant cysts, they themselves are cancerous only about 1 percent of the time. They are unique in structure in that they contain a variety of the elements of human physiology, including teeth, hair, skin, and human cells. A woman is most likely to get this type of cyst in her twenties. If they rupture, the highly toxic fluid can poison the entire system, indicating emergency treatment.

TREATMENT OPTIONS

If a cyst turns out to be one of the above three but is not malignant, the cyst alone—and not your ovary—may be removed. This can often be accomplished via the laparoscopic procedure or by a slightly more complex operation called an ovarian cystectomy, which removes the cyst without removing the ovary.

Another alternative is to drain the cyst by means of a needle inserted through the vagina. Once the fluid has been removed, the cyst collapses and fertility can be restored.

FIGHT A HYSTERECTOMY!

At no time should you consent to a hysterectomy for a nonmalignant ovarian cyst. Some surgeons may try to frighten you into this operation, claiming that it is a preventative measure against ovarian cancer later in life. Always get a second—and if necessary, a third—opinion.

The actual incidence of ovarian cancer among women in their forties and fifties is only between 1 and 2 percent. Even in the case of exceptionally large cysts, your ovaries can usually remain safely inside your body.

THE NEW TEST FOR OVARIAN CANCER

> To help rule out the possibility that an ovarian cyst is malignant, there is a new blood test called a CA 125. When used in conjunction with the pelvic sonogram, the CA 125 can rule out almost completely the possibility of malignancy. Both these tests are discussed in Chapter Seven.

IF YOUR CYST IS MALIGNANT ...

If your cysts do indicate that a clear-cut malignancy is present (and I stress *already present,* not impending), then and only then is organ removal necessary.

POLYCYSTIC OVARIAN DISEASE AND INFERTILITY

In addition to the ovarian cysts already mentioned, there is one more type that can seriously influence your reproductive health. These are the growths that develop from a condition called polycystic ovarian disease (PCO), which in its most severe form is called Stein–Leventhal syndrome, after the two men who pioneered its research.

How PCO Develops

When you have PCO, a malfunction in your body chemistry keeps your eggs from receiving the necessary growth signal from your brain. Instead of maturing and releasing, they remain inside their shell and die. When this happens, the follicles (the shell in which your egg grows) swell with fluid and develop into cysts. Each time another of your eggs is trapped in this manner, another cyst forms, until eventually your ovary is so overloaded it begins to enlarge, often becoming as big as a grapefruit.

PCO: THE SYMPTOMS

Caused by a hormone imbalance that is constant and not related to the menstrual cycle, polycystic ovarian disease can cause these symptoms:

- ◆ Menstrual irregularities
- ◆ Excess body hair
- ◆ Obesity
- ◆ Inability to conceive

How PCO Affects Fertility

PCO primarily affects fertility by inhibiting or stopping ovulation. In milder forms of the disease and in its early stages, some irregular ovulation can occur. However, in more severe cases, almost no possibility for egg release exists. When eggs become trapped in every cycle, complete infertility results.

In addition, because high levels of estrogen are also associated with PCO (thought to be caused by excess body fat converting too much of the hormone androgen into a substance called androgenous estrogen), there may be overstimulation and growth of the endometrium, or uterine lining. Since the woman is not likely to be menstruating on any kind of regular basis, the lining is not regularly shed. As a result, abnormal cell growth and even malignancy may occur.

Protecting Your Fertility from PCO

Although there is no real cure for PCO, once it has been diagnosed and treated, many patients experience a decrease in its fertility-related consequences. Certain fertility drugs—for example, clomiphene citrate (brand name, Clomid), a medication discussed later in this book—can often help stimulate egg production and encourage ovulation, allowing some PCO patients to conceive.

THREAT 5: ABORTIONS

While no surgical procedure is totally without risk, most medical experts agree that when performed properly, in a sterile, clinical environment, by a skilled physician, an abortion is safe and poses no threat to the future of your reproductive health. However, all too often, too many abortions are not performed correctly, and this is when fertility problems can arise.

HOW AN ABORTION AFFECTS YOUR FERTILITY

Although the chance that you will experience serious fertility-related damage is slim, it does exist. If your abortion is not done properly, three major consequences can result:

- ◆ A damaged cervix
- ◆ A torn uterus
- ◆ A perforated bowel

In all cases instruments involved in removing the fetus actually rip open these areas, causing hemorrhaging and making future pregnancies difficult or impossible. In addition, occasionally an abscess can form inside your abdomen as a result of the abortion. If left untreated, this can lead to PID. Also, if there are bacteria or viruses present in your vagina prior to the abortion, the procedure can exacerbate their travel to other parts of your reproductive system, also resulting in PID.

THE MORE ABORTIONS, THE GREATER THE RISKS

When they are performed correctly, it is doubtful that one or even two abortions will have negative effects on your ability to conceive in the future. However, if performed repeatedly, especially at close intervals (when used as a method of birth control, for example), the operation itself can cause a number of serious problems, some of which will place your fertility in grave danger. These include:

- *Incompetent cervix.* This occurs when, as the result of too many abortions, your cervix becomes too weak to sustain a normal pregnancy. This can place you at higher risk for miscarriage and/or premature labor.
- *Stenotic uterus.* Because scar tissue can form after every abortion, when you have too many operations, especially at close intervals, potentially dangerous adhesions can develop. When they do, your uterus can become stenotic, or "too tight" to function. Eventually it can seal shut, and all chance for pregnancy becomes impossible.
- *Damaged uterine lining.* Because an abortion involves scraping the tender uterine lining in which your fertilized egg is implanted, when the procedure is performed too often, that lining can become too thin and too weak to sustain a future embryo or nourish its growth. If you do conceive, miscarriage, birth defects, or premature labor can result.

ABORTION AND FERTILITY PROTECTION: WHAT YOU CAN DO

Although the majority of abortions performed today are safe, in the event that you find it necessary to have this procedure, there are some precautions you can take to ensure an extra measure of fertility protection:

- Refrain from sexual intercourse for at least four to six weeks following your abortion. Penetration that takes place too soon increases your risk of structural damage and infection.
- Remain on the lookout for signs of infection following your abortion:
  - severe pelvic pain
  - prolonged abdominal cramping
  - fever
  - hemorrhaging
  Although you can expect *some* bleeding for two to four weeks, it should amount to no more than a light menstrual flow.
- Receive comprehensive follow-up care. This should include administration of antibiotics for five to seven days following the abortion to help decrease the spread of potential infection.
- Be tested for sexually transmitted diseases prior to your abortion and prescribed antibiotics for seven to ten days if there is any chance you are harboring an infection.

DID A PAST ABORTION HARM YOUR FERTILITY?
HOW TO TELL

While the abortion procedure does carry some fertility-related risks, the good news is they are usually few and far between. In the unfortunate event that complications do arise, they normally do so soon (hours or days) after your abortion, when immediate treatment can usually prevent any fertility damage. That means if you suffered no postoperative problems or symptoms of infection, such as heavy bleeding or excessive pain, following your last abortion, chances are your fertility was not compromised.

If, however, problems such as a torn uterus or a perforated bowel did occur, it may be wise to have your reproductive options reviewed by a fertility specialist, especially if your abortion was recent. This can help minimize damage to your reproductive organs and increase your chances for a healthy conception in the future.

THREAT 6: THE INTRAUTERINE BIRTH CONTROL DEVICE (IUD)

When first introduced more than thirty years ago, the IUD quickly became a popular method of birth control. It was made of various materials, including copper wound wire and plastic, and available in several shapes, including the "T" and the "loop." A physician implanted it into the uterus, where it remained effective for various lengths of time, from one to several years.

Although the device seemed to work well in avoiding pregnancy, problems began to surface in 1970, when the Dalkon Shield, an IUD manufactured by the A. H. Robbins Company, was linked to an extraordinarily high incidence of PID and, consequently, infertility. The shape of this unit, which featured a long, wicklike tail, seemed to act as an inviting entryway for potentially deadly bacteria and viruses. More than 200,000 lawsuits were filed against the company from 1970 to 1974, and eventually Robbins went bankrupt. Needless to say, the Dalkon Shield was taken off the market.

Although other IUDS—the Copper T and the Lippes Loop, for example—were never proven defective, rather than push against the tide of popular opinion, their manufacturers voluntarily removed them from the market as well.

HOW AN IUD WORKS

> The latest research garnered from studies in Chile has shown that eggs recovered from women who were currently using the IUD were, for the most part, *un*fertilized. Based on this evidence, researchers now believe the IUD avoids pregnancy by incapacitating sperm. Other studies, however, continue to show it might also work by interfering with implantation.

CAN AN IUD HARM YOUR FERTILITY? HOW TO TELL

Currently there are two new types of IUDs available: the Copper T 380A, by GynoMed Pharmaceuticals, and Progestasert, by the Alza Corporation. As effective as these units have proved to be, for some women they might still pose a problem.

When an IUD is in place, it makes your uterus more vulnerable to infection by allowing for easier passage of bacteria into your system. If you should have sex with an infected partner or if you are exposed to certain bacteria in other circumstances (both of which are fully explained in Chapter Four), an IUD can be a hazard. This is especially true if you are under age twenty-five, since your cervix normally remains partially open until your middle twenties.

In addition, an IUD can also be a problem if you have a history of sexually transmitted diseases or PID. Studies show an IUD may increase your odds for contracting them again, especially if you are sexually active and have a number of partners. Because both of these conditions can cause scar tissue in your reproductive tract each time they occur, each incidence can add to your risk of infertility.

For these reasons, I generally do not believe an IUD should be pre-scribed for any woman who has not yet completed her family, unless certain circumstances prevail. If you and your doctor mutually decide that an IUD is the only reasonable birth control option for you, you must remain critically aware of any signs of impending problems and seek medical attention immediately. This would include any signs or symp-toms of STDs and any that could indicate a possible problem, including pelvic pain, irregular bleeding, unusual discharge, or persistent fever.

If any of these signs appear, see your doctor immediately for a com-plete pelvic evaluation, consider having your IUD removed, and make certain antibiotic treatment is started immediately.

IF YOUR IUD HAS ALREADY CAUSED HARM— WHAT TO DO NOW

If you had an IUD in the past and you experienced no problems, then it is likely your fertility was not harmed. In fact, studies show that the most likely threats occur *only* in the first three months following insertion, when, it is believed, sexually transmitted bacteria already present in your vagina may be pushed up into the uterus. After four months' time, your IUD–PID related risks are equal to that of women who do not use any form of contraception. So if you did not experience any problems while your IUD was in place, your fertility is probably in good shape now.

However, if you did undergo some complications, especially if you experienced pain, spotting, or heavy bleeding, and you did not see a doctor, it's possible you may have contracted an infection that caused some damage to your reproductive organs. In this case, a hystero-salpingogram, an x-ray of the uterus and tubes, or a laparoscopy may be in order to ensure that you are problem-free.

THREAT 7: ECTOPIC PREGNANCY

In an ectopic pregnancy, some biological malfunction keeps your fertilized egg from reaching your uterus. Instead, it implants itself some-where else in your body, such as your abdomen, on your ovary, or, most commonly, in your fallopian tube, and starts to grow. When this occurs, your conception cannot survive.

In the past it was believed only one out of every 200 pregnancies was ectopic. The American College of Obstetrics and Gynecology suggests that the present ratio is one out of every 100—possibly due to the concurrent rise in PID, damage from which is thought to be the leading cause of ectopic pregnancy.

Complications stemming from ectopic pregnancy are currently the leading cause of maternal death.

HOW ECTOPIC PREGNANCIES HARM YOUR FERTILITY

Because most ectopic pregnancies take root in your fallopian tubes, the space in which your fetus can grow is severely limited. However, not realizing it is somewhere out of your uterus, it begins to develop normally, expanding at a fairly rapid rate.

Once the fetus starts developing, it isn't long before your embryo is straining against the sides of the tube. If left untreated, the tube can rupture, causing severe damage and potentially fatal hemorrhaging.

Although you can still conceive with only one fallopian tube, ectopic pregnancies are likely to recur, so it's highly possible that both tubes can be destroyed within a relatively short period of time, canceling all chances for natural conception.

In addition, even if your ectopic pregnancy is removed in time, scar tissue may result, inhibiting or even blocking both sperm passage and egg transport.

ARE YOU AT RISK?

One of the most unfortunate aspects of ectopic pregnancy is that it can strike any woman at any time. However, there are *some* factors that can place you at a higher than average risk:

- A history of PID
- IUD use (which leads to PID)
- Previous ectopic pregnancy
- Endometriosis
- Tubal sterilization
- Pregnancy over age thirty-five
- Two or more abortions
- Heavy smoking
- Progesterone only (mini-pill)
- Your mother took diethylstibestrol (DES)

THE SYMPTOMS

One of the most devastating aspects of ectopic pregnancy is that, in the beginning, your conception appears to be normal. A pregnancy blood test will read positive, with no qualifying factors, and because your conception was, from a fertilization standpoint, successful, you will *feel* pregnant and have all the physical symptoms. However, an ectopic pregnancy is *not* normal, so as your baby begins to grow, distinct signs will appear:

- Abdominal tenderness
- Lower abdominal pain on both sides or on the side opposite your egg's site of implantation
- Pain in your shoulder (caused by bleeding into your abdomen)
- Dizziness
- Fainting
- Urge to defecate

If your abdominal pain becomes severe or if you experience a sudden and overwhelming cramping, seek emergency medical treatment *immediately*. These may be signs that your tube is starting to rupture.

PROTECTING YOUR FERTILITY: WHAT YOU CAN DO

There is no way to *stop* an ectopic pregnancy, but if you are at high risk for this problem, a hysterosalpingogram—an x-ray of your fallopian tubes—can help show whether there is a blockage capable of stopping egg transport. If a blockage is discovered, a laparoscopy or other surgical procedure can be performed to help clear your tubes before you conceive again. This can substantially reduce your risk of another ectopic pregnancy and thereby increase your fertility.

EARLY DIAGNOSIS: ANOTHER WAY TO PROTECT YOUR FERTILITY

Even if you are not considered at high risk for an ectopic pregnancy there is no way to guarantee your conception will not be out of womb. Conversely, even if you are at high risk, your pregnancy could be normal. For this reason I strongly advise every woman to have an early sonogram, which is one of the best ways to diagnose an ectopic pregnancy. Although your doctor will rarely be able to see your actual pregnancy at a very early stage, what he/she can detect is whether your pregnancy sac is somewhere outside your uterus. This is especially important if your pregnancy is in your tubes, since the earlier this problem is diagnosed, the better your chance of avoiding a potentially fatal tubal rupture.

In addition, the development of ultrasensitive human chorionic gonadotropin (hCG) pregnancy blood tests have also proved to be a major advancement in early diagnosis of this pregnancy trauma. Whereas diagnosis once required that a pregnancy be in its eighth to tenth week, now, by combining the results of the hCG tests and an ultrasonogram, correct diagnosis can often be made just four to six weeks after conception.

IF AN ECTOPIC PREGNANCY IS DIAGNOSED . . .

Should your doctor diagnose an ectopic pregnancy, you will need a laparoscopy, a relatively simple surgical procedure (see Chapters Seven and Sixteen), or a laparotomy, a slightly more complex procedure. The purpose is to remove the ectopic pregnancy.

If an unruptured tubal pregnancy is diagnosed, the most common treatment is a salpingostomy (performed during a laparoscopy or laparotomy), in which an incision is made into the wall of the fallopian tube directly over the site of the pregnancy, and the conceptus is removed.

To help safeguard against future infections that can lead to PID, as well as against additional ectopic pregnancies, your doctor should prescribe an antibiotic as soon as your ectopic pregnancy is diagnosed and add 100 to 200 milliliters (ml) of dextran 70 (brand name Hyskon) to your peritoneal cavity (the area surrounding your fallopian tube) as soon as removal is completed. If your blood type is Rh negative, you should receive a RhoGAM injection immediately after the procedure (see Chapter Twelve).

THE CONTROVERSIAL NEW TREATMENT FOR ECTOPIC PREGNANCY

Recently researchers have begun to experiment with the use of chemotherapeutic agents (the drugs used to kill cancer cells) as a way of treating ectopic pregnancy. At present the treatment is still somewhat controversial, but many believe it can be advantageous in treating ectopics that are very small or those that occur in the wall of the uterus. Further studies are needed to determine if this method is indeed safe and effective.

A FINAL THOUGHT ABOUT YOUR FERTILITY

Although anything that has the potential to harm your fertility is a threat that should be taken seriously, it's also important to realize that in many instances fertility problems can be prevented or damage minimized by early treatment. Use the information in this chapter to learn more about your body—and your fertility—and to protect against complications. Use it, too, to help find a doctor who will be your partner and treat you with the respect and care you deserve.

· 3 ·

FINALLY! THE TRUTH ABOUT MALE FERTILITY

Although it took a long time for a man's reproductive system to be viewed with the same scrutiny as a woman's, fortunately a double standard in this area of medicine no longer exists. Today we have a more complete understanding of conception, including how, why, and *how often* male fertility problems can occur. The truth of the matter is this:

- ◆ 40 to 50 percent of all conception problems are male related.

PLUS

- ◆ Factors in the male partner's body can be directly responsible for miscarriage, premature labor, congenital malformations (birth defects), and infant death.

Another important truth: fertility is no longer just a woman's concern. Getting pregnant is a responsibility equally shared by both partners.

Perhaps even more significant, we now know that, much the way a woman can protect her fertility, so a man can protect his. Not only are there things a man can do to ensure his reproductive health, there are things he *must* do if his fertility (and his sexual vitality) are to remain active throughout his life. In fact, by simply learning what can influence the fate and future of his reproductive health, a man can learn to influence and control his childbearing options in ways never before possible!

MALE INFERTILITY:
A PROBLEM WITHIN A PROBLEM

Although new research has made it quite simple for a man to accomplish all this, in many ways protecting and ultimately treating male fertility is far more difficult than it has to be—simply because of the way men feel about the subject. Age, race, color, occupation, location, education, financial bracket—it doesn't matter. Most men still react with explosive sensitivity to even the suggestion that their fertility is not omnipotent, and the reaction invariably grows stronger if and when a problem *is* suspected.

I have, in fact, spent many hours counseling and even consoling infertility patients after their otherwise intelligent and gentle partners left our clinic in a stormy fit of temper simply because we asked them to take a sperm count. A few became verbally abusive or even physically violent toward their spouses and, on rare occasions, even to our staff.

Regardless of how your partner reacts, however, it's vital to you both that he understand his new role in the conception and delivery of a healthy baby, and the ways in which he must begin to protect his fertility right now. I believe you can help him accomplish this by sharing this chapter with him.

UNDERSTANDING A MAN'S FERTILITY

As in the case of a woman's body, a man's body requires the activity of reproductive hormones to put fertility in motion. Not coincidentally, the hormones needed to stimulate sperm production in a man are the very same substances that stimulate egg growth in a woman, FSH and LH. As in a woman's body, they are regulated and secreted into the bloodstream by the hypothalamus and pituitary glands, both of which are located in the brain. Unlike a woman, however, whose hormone levels constantly rise and fall, a man has a constant level of these biochemicals surging through his body at all times, from puberty onward. This is one of the reasons he is continually fertile every day of every month and has no time limit on his childbearing years.

HOW SPERM IS MADE

In a man's body, the main goal of both FSH and LH is to continually stimulate the production of testosterone, the male hormone manufactured in the tissue of the testicles. Found in a woman's body in tiny amounts but in a man's body in massive amounts, this hormone allows the testicles to manufacture sperm, and must remain at constant levels in order to keep production lags from occurring. Providing testosterone levels remain high, sperm cells are continually manufactured with production-line speed, twenty-four hours a day, from puberty onward.

FROM TESTICLES TO PENIS: HOW SPERM GETS TO YOU

Once manufactured, the sperm must be allowed to mature, travel unhampered from the testicles to the penis, and then be forcefully ejaculated *if* the male fertility cycle is to be completed. To help the sperm do that, five other equally important organs, glands, and vessels make up the remainder of a man's reproductive system:

- *The epididymis.* Two twenty-one-foot-long tubes coiled into an area just one-and-one-half inches wide, they sit atop each testicle inside the scrotal sac. Each sperm cell spends about twelve days passing through this structure, where it undergoes a maturing process that includes learning to swim. (This ensures that it can navigate through a woman's reproductive system and reach her egg.)
- *The vas deferens.* This consists of two thick tubelike structures that extend from the top of each epididymis through the scrotum (the loose skin sac surrounding the testicles) up into the abdomen, where it passes down into the bottom of the prostate gland and eventually empties into the urethra. Their main purpose is to transport the sperm.
- *Seminal vesicles.* These are two small glands located just below the bladder that secrete fructose, a vital component of semen, the ejaculatory fluid that helps transport the sperm into a woman's reproductive system.
- *The prostate.* This gland also secretes ejaculatory fluid and helps sperm achieve their final maturation and an increase in potency.
- *The urethra.* This is a long narrow duct that runs from just above the top of the penis down through the shaft to the tip. It transports sperm out of the body.

HOW SEX MAKES IT ALL WORK

Although a man has a constant supply of sperm ready to be ejaculated at all times, he still needs one more signal before this process can begin. This one he receives from his partner, in the form of sexual stimulation.

Unlike a woman's body, which does not need to be sexually stimulated in order for conception to occur, a man must undergo the excitement phase, including a penile erection, to give his sperm the "go" signal. Once he is excited, the delicate nerve endings in his penis send messages throughout his reproductive system to create the power necessary to transport sperm and forcefully ejaculate it. The biological sequence of events goes somewhat like this:

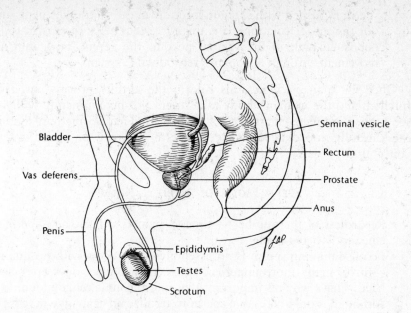

Bladder

Vas deferens

Penis

Epididymis

Testes

Scrotum

Seminal vesicle

Rectum

Prostate

Anus

The Male Reproductive System

Sperm is manufactured in the testes (or testicles) and then spends about twelve days passing through the epididymis, a twenty-one-foot-long coiled tube that sits inside the scrotal sac. It then passes through the vas deferens, a long, tubelike structure that winds through the abdomen, past the prostate gland, and eventually connects to the urethra, a long hollow tube inside the shaft of the penis. As sperm passes through the vas deferens, the seminal vesicles and the prostate both secrete fluid that aids in propelling the sperm toward the penis. Sexual stimulation, leading to orgasm, is the mechanism that pumps the sperm and the fluid through the penis, shooting it from the man's body with shotgun force into the woman's body. Once inside, the sperm navigate through a woman's reproductive system until they reach her egg and—hopefully—fertilization occurs.

1. As sexual arousal occurs, a man's penis becomes erect. This sends a signal to the vas deferens to begin a series of rapid muscular contractions.
2. Once this movement begins, the sperm is pumped forward, from the epididymis and the ampullae (a depotlike area in which some sperm is stored) through the entire vas deferens.
3. As the sperm travels, it passes by the seminal vesicles, where a fructose solution is secreted to help push it toward the prostate gland, where more fluid is collected. Since all this seminal fluid is actually secreted behind the sperm as it passes, the first squirt of an ejaculation is always the most potent.
4. Once past the prostate, the sperm is transported into the base of the urethra, just above the top of the penis, to wait for its final release signal, the intense, rhythmic muscular contraction of orgasm.
5. The moment orgasm begins, it creates a power so strong that the

sperm is pushed with shotgun force down the shaft of the penis and out the tip (ejaculation). It is this force that helps the sperm to be deposited high in the vagina, next to the cervix, facilitating its movement through a woman's reproductive system.

Once the man ejaculates, his role in the fertility process has been fulfilled, and the woman's body takes over. Nowhere in nature will you see a more complete "marriage" of the male and female anatomy than in the carefully coordinated dance of sperm and egg on their way to conception.

SPERM FACTS YOU NEED TO KNOW

- ◆ Regardless of the number of times a man ejaculates, new sperm is constantly being made.
- ◆ Because making sperm is an assembly-line process with no quality control, many more imperfect sperm than perfect ones are ejaculated. That's why it's important that sperm counts remain high.
- ◆ Although it only takes one sperm to fertilize an egg, anywhere from 20 million to 200 million sperm can be ejected during an ejaculation. Because of a series of natural barriers in the female reproductive system, however, only about forty of those sperm will ever reach the vicinity of an egg.
- ◆ Since very few barriers exist in a laboratory conception (like in vitro fertilization), they can sometimes be used to help men with sperm counts under 5 million per cubic centimeter (cc, about a drop of semen).
- ◆ While semen is necessary to propel sperm into a woman's body, the size of an ejaculation in no way reflects the number of sperm a man is producing. Sterile men can produce a tablespoon or more of semen, while highly potent men may ejaculate only a few drops. However, insufficient amounts of semen could mean the sperm never reach the egg. What's the average ejaculation? From 2.5 to 5.0 cc (5.5 cc equals 1 teaspoon).
- ◆ A high sperm count doesn't always ensure conception, and a low sperm count doesn't always mean failure. Nature can take some surprising twists and turns, and the long shot can become the winner.

WHAT CAN HARM A MAN'S FERTILITY

The sperm-making process is a delicate and complex biological one that can be overturned, we now know, by a variety of different factors. Since each step in the sperm's journey is a vital one, anything that inhibits or blocks its activity at any stage, from manufacturing to ejaculation, has the potential to harm male fertility. What can make a difference?

* Any activity that can injure the reproductive organs
* Bacteria, viruses, or other microorganisms that can hamper organ function or sperm manufacture or transport
* The development of scar tissue as a result of disease or infection

HERE'S THE GOOD NEWS!

While there are a few villains over which there is no control (congenital malformations of the genitals, for example, where a man is born without testicles), the good news is that, for the most part, most men do have at least *some* power over the factors that can affect them. To exert that power, a man need only become aware of *what* can harm him and then build a few basic precautions into the course of his daily living.

THE FORCES THAT ZAP A MAN'S FERTILITY: WHAT HE NEEDS TO KNOW RIGHT NOW!

THREAT 1: THE MUMPS

One of the most common of all childhood diseases is the mumps, a viral infection that attacks the lymph glands, which are located throughout the body, including the groin. Contracting mumps before puberty carries no specific fertility-related danger, but that changes for a man once adulthood arrives. What can happen when a grown man catches mumps?

* The virus can invade his testicles, causing pain and swelling.
* His testicles can lose their ability to make sperm for a few weeks or even permanently.

Very often the end result of adult-onset mumps is permanent infertility.

Mumps: Is He at Risk?

Having mumps in childhood provides a man with lifetime immunity. Because, however, an accurate diagnosis is not always made, a man may believe he has protection from this virus when in fact he does not.

The problem stems from the fact that the symptoms of mumps (most especially swelling of the testicles) can overlap with those caused by mononucleosis, and a testicle problem called "torsion." Only a physician, who can rely on blood tests and a physical exam, can make an accurate diagnosis. Since, however, childhood diseases often come and go with only a parental diagnosis to confirm them, in the case of mumps, a misdiagnosis is too often made. The end result: mumps may never have actually occurred. This is why I routinely tell each patient's husband that unless he is 100 percent certain he has had the mumps (checking with his own pediatrician if possible), he should stay away from anyone who has the disease, including his own children. This is especially important during the very early stages of the disease, when transmission factors are the highest. If exposure does occur, a man should seek immediate medical attention.

ADULT MUMPS: A NEW WARNING!

Even though a highly effective mumps vaccine has been available since 1967, the U.S. Food and Drug Administration (FDA) recently announced that more and more young (unvaccinated) adults are coming down with the disease. The FDA advises that both men and women born after 1956 make a point of discovering if they had mumps, and if they have not had it, they should ask their doctor about a vaccine. A man exposed to the mumps virus should seek medical treatment immediately, especially if the following symptoms appear:

◆ Low-grade fever
◆ Swelling in neck, underarm, or groin glands
◆ Mild sore throat
◆ Achy, flulike feeling

If mumps is diagnosed, he should seek immediate treatment from a urologist or a fertility specialist and keep a close check on his sperm count until levels return to normal.

THREAT 2: SPORTS TRAUMAS

More than ever, fitness is a part of everyone's life. However, as wholesome as being physically active is, it can harm fertility. How? Through sports-related genital trauma, accidents that can damage or even permanently impair a man's reproductive system.

What Can Harm Him the Most

Although a genital trauma can come from almost any activity, the most common cause is a team sport:

◆ Football   ◆ Basketball
◆ Hockey   ◆ Baseball
◆ Soccer

However, a man can also get hurt during one-on-one competitions like tennis or racquetball, where the speed and impact of the ball itself can completely shatter a testicle, or even when engaged in solo activities. Accidents occurring during bicycling and horseback riding, for example, have been responsible for some of the most traumatic of all genital injuries.

What Happens When a Man Gets Hurt

Although the type of sport a man is playing largely determines the type of injury he can sustain, certain types of traumas tend to be more common than others:

- *Ruptured epididymis.* Damage here can keep sperm from maturing enough to fertilize an egg.
- *A split or torn vas deferens.* Damage can act much like a vasectomy and stop sperm transport.
- *Shattered testicles.* This not only destroys sperm production, but also ends the ability to manufacture the important male hormone testosterone.
- *Injured seminal vesicles and/or prostate gland.* Since both these organs supply seminal fluid, damage can lead to ejaculatory problems that could keep sperm from leaving the body.
- *Bladder damage.* This could harm the delicate muscle structure that keeps sperm from mixing with urine and urine from leaking into the urethra and damaging sperm.
- *Back trauma.* In the case of a slipped disk or a spinal chord injury, for example, nerves controlling erection or other actions of the male reproductive system may be severed or damaged.

CAN A PENIS BREAK?

Although every part of a man's reproductive system is subject to destruction from injury or disease, one of the most resilient organs—and the one least likely to be affected—is the penis. Comprised of exceptionally strong muscle and tissue, it can't break and usually rebounds from injury quite rapidly.

Biker's Impotence: A New Discovery

A brand-new study from the University of Southern California School of Medicine shows that a serious cyclist might be placing his fertility in extreme danger. How? According to Harin Padma-Nathan, assistant professor of urology at USC and a specialist in sexual disorders, many of his male patients suffering from impotence had one important factor in common: they all rode their bicycles at least 100 miles a week. The problem? Repeated thrusting on the pedals was causing a banging of the groin against the bicycle seat, damaging critical arteries and nerves. The danger was increased when riders used a hard, narrow seat and maintained an aggressive riding style for long periods of time. A lean body also seemed to contribute to the problem.

To help ensure his fertility, every man who regularly rides a bicycle should remain critically aware of the following warning signs of biker's impotence:

- ◆ Numbness in the backside
- ◆ Difficulty in getting an erection after biking, or for one or two days that follow
- ◆ Pain in the genital area

If any of these symptoms appear after biking and last longer than two days, a man should see a doctor immediately.

To help keep problems from occurring, Professor Padma-Nathan recommends the following precautions:

- ◆ Periodically pull your body up from the bike seat when riding long distances.
- ◆ Position the bike seat so that body weight does not shift on the downstroke.

It is also important to note that damage from biker's impotence is cumulative. Without treatment, this temporary problem could become permanent.

Protection Against All Sporting Injuries

Because nearly every sporting activity has the potential for genital harm, any man who is athletically active must use adequate protective equipment, even when the possibilities for problems are slim. Many men seem to eschew this thought of sports protection, believing it's only for "wimps," but I can't express strongly enough the importance of safeguarding the genitals, especially in amateur sports. In fact, so important is the concept of adequate protection that in professional sports today team physicians, managers, and even the players themselves are actively campaigning for more stringent regulations regarding the mandatory use of protective gear during all types of sporting games.

SPORTS INJURIES: WHO'S AT HIGH RISK?

Since the risk of injury increases when players are less experienced, the most serious accidents can and often do happen to young, amateur athletes, men in their early to mid-twenties. Many won't realize until they try to have a child, and can't, sometimes ten or fifteen years later, just how important having that protection would have been. Every man who participates in sports must use protection, the best he can afford, including:

- Penile cups
- Jock straps
- Padded genital protector
- Sturdy protective clothing

All these items can make a big difference in protecting the priceless commodity of reproductive health.

What to Do If an Injury Does Occur

Even when protection is used, and certainly when it is not, the risk of sports-related genital injury still exists. To ensure that his fertility and his reproductive organs remain in good health, a man must also take some important self-care steps should an injury be sustained—steps that could make a difference between damage that is temporary and that which is permanent:

1. Seek *immediate* emergency medical treatment. Many men believe it is macho to suffer in silence, but getting no treatment or waiting too long can be disastrous. When genital traumas are treated early enough, damage to reproductive health can be greatly minimized.
2. Seek follow-up care. Even if emergency treatment is received, follow-up visits with a urologist, the type of physician who generally specializes in male fertility, can help minimize damage and monitor the healing process.
3. Check sperm count. Although sperm count can remain low for several weeks or even months following an injury, it should rise

again if the damage was not permanent. Checking sperm count periodically until that rise occurs can facilitate getting additional medical care if needed.

THREAT 3: FITNESS WORKOUTS

Although a man seldom experiences genital injury while jogging or doing aerobic exercise, there is some evidence that some fitness activities can affect fertility by altering the temperature of the testicles and thus hampering sperm movement and production.

Too Hot to Make a Baby!

In order for a man's testicles to function at peak efficiency, their temperature must remain between 94 and 96 degrees Fahrenheit, approximately two to four degrees cooler than normal body temperature. To help maintain the correct temperature, and ensure fertility, nature placed the testicles outside the body and equipped them with a special set of muscles that draw them close to the body when they get too cold and drop them loose when the temperature rises too high.

Sometimes, however, certain activities temporarily override this natural reaction and allow the temperature of the testicles to rise too high. When this occurs, sperm production stops or significantly decreases. In addition, there is some evidence that prolonged exposure to high body heat may also affect the epididymis, the organ where sperm mature and learn to swim. This can affect a man's immediate ability to conceive a child and sometimes results in permanent sterility. A defective epididymis can also increase the risk of miscarriage and/or birth defects by allowing greater numbers of abnormal sperm to be produced.

Since certain fitness activities can and usually do increase overall body temperature, sometimes they can affect fertility as well. Fortunately, for most men, once the body cools, any sperm production that *was* disrupted returns to normal. However, for those who have a borderline low sperm count or testicles that are already too hot due to certain vascular problems (discussed later in this book) fertility may be further affected by the choice of activity.

The Workouts That Can Affect His Fertility

While any activity that substantially raises body heat has the potential to affect sperm count and motility, the following fitness workouts are thought to bring about the most temperature-related problems in the least amount of time:

- Rowing machines
- Simulated cross-country ski machines
- Treadmills
- Duration aerobics
- Repetitive calisthenics and/or aerobics
- Jogging

In addition, *any* exercise can be made more hazardous when certain workout clothes are worn, primarily those that hold in body heat. These include

- Exceptionally tight shorts
- Synthetic fabrics that don't breathe
- Tight-fitting jeans (worn right after working out)
- Tight bikini underwear

Good News

Fortunately, the solution to any of these problems is simple. A man doesn't have to stop working out—as long as he makes sure his testicles remain free enough to pull away from his body when temperatures get too hot. The avoidance of tight underwear when working out and tight jeans afterward could be all his body needs to ensure a high sperm count and steady production.

In addition, he should try to spend time aerating his genitals, by removing all clothing from his lower body and covering himself with just a light robe or a towel wrap after exercising. This can go a long way toward helping his genitals recover from heat buildup and constriction.

Health Club Fertility Hazards

In addition to the workout, some of the perks provided by health clubs can affect male fertility by further increasing the temperature of testicles. If you are trying to conceive, your partner should avoid

- Saunas
- Steam baths
- Hot tubs
- Extra hot showers

These can be especially hazardous directly after vigorous exercise, when body heat can rise to a point that is dangerous to sperm.

THREAT 4: STRESS

Interesting new research has brought to light evidence linking stress to fertility—and especially to infertility—not only in women, but in men. While we previously believed the only link between stress and male fertility occurred when tension reduced a man's ability to have an erection, we now know that stress can affect his reproductive system in a variety of ways.

In recent studies by the Department of Physiology at the Medical College of Ohio in Toledo, the following facts were learned:

◆ Both a man's autonomic nervous sytem and his adrenal hormones actively participate in the stress response, and changes in these areas can impede sperm production and release.
◆ Emotional stress can depress testosterone levels and thus interfere with sperm production.
◆ In animal studies it was learned that, in addition to stress, high altitudes, surgery, and immobilization affect testosterone levels and mating behavior, with varying effects on the testicles.
◆ Extreme tension and fatigue for prolonged periods of time do lead to psychological impotence. This in turn often leads to more worry (about the impotence itself), which in turn can add enough stress to affect the hypothalamus gland, alter levels of FSH and LH, and ultimately lower both testosterone levels and sperm count.

In addition, many independent studies have shown that even minimal stress has the ability to cause a man's sperm count to drop unexplainably. The greater and more prolonged the stress becomes, the more serious the damage that can occur.

The Good News!

As devastating as stress can be on a man's fertility, the good news is that effects are usually only temporary, lessening and even disappearing completely when the stressful situation is resolved. In addition, researchers believe, by keeping stress levels under control (especially by *not worrying* about temporary bouts with impotence), a man can give himself a good measure of fertility protection as well as a boost to his sex life!

THREAT 5: COLDS, THE FLU, AND OTHER DISEASES

In much the same way that a woman's menstrual cycle can be affected by changes in her body chemistry, so can a man's sperm-making abilities be jeopardized if something causes his white blood cell count to rise.

When it does, the result can be a bout of infertility lasting anywhere from several days to several months or even longer.

What kinds of health problems can cause this temporary effect on a man's fertility?

♦ The flu	♦ An acne flare-up
♦ Diarrhea	♦ An abscessed tooth
♦ A bacterial infection	♦ Mononucleosis
♦ A virus	♦ Epstein–Barr virus

Naturally, this doesn't mean that a man with a cold can't make you pregnant. Of course, he can! But depending on the strength of his immune system, a man's fertility is at least somewhat compromised every time he gets sick.

The Infections That Can Harm His Fertility

In addition to those problems that can temporarily cause a man's sperm count to suffer, there are some diseases, as well as some infections of the reproductive tract itself, that can have a more powerful and long-lasting effect on his fertility:

- *Urethritis,* an inflammation of the tube that carries sperm from his body
- *Epididymitis,* an infection of the epididymis, which can affect sperm maturation and transport
- *Prostatitis,* an infection of the prostate gland, which can affect sperm motility and cause impotence and ejaculatory problems

When left untreated, any of these infections can partially or even completely destroy a man's reproductive organs, rendering him permanently infertile.

The Good News!

Although almost any bacteria or viruses that invade a man's body can settle in his reproductive tract and cause one or more of these problems, the culprits are most often the microrganisms associated with STDs. You'll learn how and why they occur (and what you and your partner can do to protect fertility) in Chapter Four. Right now, the good news to remember is that, caught early, nearly all of these infections can be easily cured using a simple antibiotic regimen for just seven to ten days.

To help ensure that he does receive that all-important early treatment, a man should remain critically aware of any of the following symptoms and report them to his doctor immediately:

- Infection, especially in the penis
- Pain, anywhere in the genital area
- Genital swelling
- Difficulty in urinating, including a burning sensation
- General genital sensitivity or discomfort
- Fatigue
- Low-grade fever
- General feeling of malaise
- Inability to father a child, especially if his partner's fertility tests okay.

DIABETES AND A MAN'S FERTILITY

One of the most physically threatening conditions is diabetes, when the biochemistry needed for the proper metabolization of sugars and simple carbohydrates is somehow disrupted. A diabetic man can suffer ejaculatory and/or potency-related problems. These difficulties can usually be controlled when the diabetes is treated, so it's imperative that a man be checked for this disease if he has any of the following symptoms:

- Excessive thirst
- Craving for sweets
- Excessive urination

Because diabetes can be hereditary, he should also be checked regularly (via a simple urine and/or blood test) if any close family members have had this disease.

A WORD ABOUT SEX AND MALE FERTILITY

While the male genitalia are built to endure both the friction and thrusting of even the most active intercourse, there are times when sex can get too rough:

- If testicles are squeezed too hard or subjected to weighted pressure for a prolonged period of time, damage to the epididymis as well as the testicles can occur.
- Oral sex performed too vigorously can cause some trauma and bruising that could have residual effects on a man's ability to make sperm for up to several weeks.
- The sharp plastic edges and/or the "tails" of certain IUDs can make

contact with the penis during heavy or deep thrusting and cause some inflammation and/or localized trauma or bleeding. This is even more likely if a man is uncircumcised: his foreskin can be ripped or torn during especially deep intercourse.

Although no permanent damage usually ensues from any of these activities, if bleeding occurs and/or persists even after pressure is applied and/or if localized infection sets in, a man should seek medical treatment as soon as possible to ensure that no harmful bacteria invade the urethra.

In addition, if a man experiences any unusual pain or discomfort in his penis, testicles, or general genital area during sex, he should seek medical treatment immediately. As in the case with women, painful intercourse for men is a sign that medical attention is needed.

SEX TOYS AND MALE FERTILITY

In addition to rough sex, some sex toys or aids, such as penile rings and vibrators, can, when used in a rough or vigorous manner, produce trauma to the male genitals and have some effects on fertility. I heard about a couple in France who, during a particularly vigorous sexual encounter, were worked into such a frenzy that they didn't notice that the electric massager the woman was using had begun to short out. When she reached down to touch her partner's genitals, he received a shock of enough impact to destroy his epididymis and all future sperm production. That was, of course, an uncommon injury (most vibrators today are battery operated and shockproof); still, it shows that whenever the genitals are involved, precautions must be taken to protect them.

FERTILITY TESTS

While it is immeasurably important that a man continually monitor his own health for the signs and symptoms of fertility-robbing conditions, self-care alone is not enough. Although there is no equivalent of the gyn exam for men, every man should undergo at least one yearly physical. For optimum fertility protection and care, the examination should include the following areas:

THE TESTICLES

The most vital of the male reproductive organs, they should be carefully examined regularly by the man himself, as well as by his physican, for

- ◆ Lumps
- ◆ Tenderness

* Discoloration
* Swelling
* Rigidity of the testicles themselves or in the
  surrounding scrotal sac and/or genital area

Not only can these be signs of genital infections, they can also signal testicle cancer, a growing concern for men of all ages.

THE PENIS

The penis should be checked for these signs:

* Discoloration
* Growths
* Lesions
* Blisters
* Warts
* Abnormal discharge

The doctor should gently squeeze the tip of the penis to see if any abnormal discharge is emitted; if there is, a urethra culture might help track down the presence of harmful bacteria or viruses.

CURRENT SEXUAL HEALTH HISTORY

Every physical should include a detailed history of any sexual malfunctions, including:

* Inability to have an erection
* Loss of sexual desire
* Inability to maintain an erection
* Premature or no ejaculation
* Pain during intercourse or any sex-related activity

Any or all of these problems could be symptoms of underlying physical problems, many of which can be related to fertility-robbing diseases or conditions.

A CHECK FOR HERNIAS AND UNDESCENDED TESTICLES

Although a hernia itself is not a direct cause of infertility, tearing of the abdominal tissue can cause a decrease in the blood supply to the vas deferens, possibly with long-term effects on the functioning of this organ.

Because surgery to repair a hernia and the procedure to correct the congenital malformation known as undescended testicles are both done very close to the spermatic cord, the blood supply to the testicles can be endangered during these operations. If the blood supply is inadvertently cut off, the testicle will atrophy and die, along with any chance for future sperm production. Only a sperm count immediately following hernia repair surgery can alert the physician to this mishap. If the count is low and does not return to normal within a few weeks' time, a second surgical procedure might be needed to restore blood flow to the testicles. This can sometimes keep permanent damage from occurring.

HIGH BLOOD PRESSURE AND DIABETES

Although high blood pressure will affect neither sperm production nor movement, some of the medications for this condition can have a negative effect on fertility. Catching and treating high blood pressure early on, preventing the need for antihypertensive medication, can be beneficial to fertility in the long run.

As previously noted, diabetes can have direct and devastating effects on a man's reproductive system, so early diagnosis and treatment can help preserve fertility, as well as general health.

A FINAL WORD ABOUT MALE FERTILITY

As medical science continues to learn about the male reproductive system, one point becomes increasingly clear: a man's fertility *cannot* be taken for granted.

THE SHOCKING TRUTH: IN THE PAST TWENTY YEARS ALONE, THE AVERAGE SPERM COUNT FOR HEALTHY COLLEGE MEN HAS DROPPED FROM 60 MILLION TO 40 MILLION PER CC OF EJACULATE.

Researchers speculate that increasing levels of stress, the proliferation of sexually transmitted diseases, wider use of alcohol, drugs, and tobacco, and exposure to radiation and other toxic substances have all contributed to this statistic. Unless men start taking steps to protect their reproductive health, these numbers can drop even further, and the incidence of male infertility can reach an all-time high. If we are to alter these statistics significantly in the next generation, the men of today must set an example for the men of tomorrow. Young boys need to be taught fertility protection at an early age—in school, on the radio and TV, in books, and, most important, by the examples set by both parents. Seeing us taking care of our reproductive health, our children will learn to do the same.

· 4 ·

SEX AND INFERTILITY
What Every Couple Needs to Know Right Now

"It can't be—I'm married. How could this happen?"

Kiersten, lawyer

"There must be a mistake. I don't hang around with 'those' kind of men."

Jennifer, health club instructor

"What? No way! My partner and I are completely faithful."

Roger, computer programmer

What are these men and women so surprised about? They've learned they have a sexually transmitted disease (STD), infections caused by a series of rapidly spreading bacteria or viruses that are usually passed on during sexual intercourse. This year alone it is estimated more than 3 million people will contract one or more STD. Many won't even know it. What is most alarming, the latest studies show that, left untreated, STDs are the leading cause of infertility in the United States today, for men as well as for women.

THE GOOD NEWS

As frustrating and damaging as STDs can be, there is good news. Once diagnosed, especially in their early stages, treatment is fast, painless, and

54

easy, and most often a complete cure can be had in just a matter of days via a simple regimen of antibiotics, eliminating nearly all threats to fertility. To accomplish this, however, you must learn the important signs and symptoms of these diseases, as well as the lifestyles and other health factors that may place you at high risk. With this information, you and your partner can protect your fertility and your sex life throughout your childbearing years.

STDs: WHAT ARE THEY? WHO'S AT RISK?

Medically speaking, a sexually transmitted disease is any of a number of infections that develop in your body primarily as the result of a sexual encounter with an infected partner. Currently, the most common STDs are these:

- ◆ Chlamydia   ◆ Gonorrhea
- ◆ Syphilis   ◆ T-mycoplasma
- ◆ Herpes   ◆ AIDS
- ◆ Human papilloma virus (HPV), which causes condoloma acuminata, or venereal warts

Because they can be transmitted during sex, some physicians now also classify three forms of vaginitis as STDs:

- ◆ Candidiasis (yeast infection)
- ◆ Trichomoniasis
- ◆ Gardnerella

While not all of these organisms can lead to infertility, if left untreated they can contribute to your inability to deliver a healthy child, as well as impair your sex life. For this reason it's imperative that you don't overlook any of the symptoms of these diseases or underestimate your chances for infection.

HOW STDs ARE SPREAD

Contrary to popular belief, STDs are not confined to those who have a wildly active sex life. Although the risks increase with the number of sexual partners you have, it's just as easy to catch an STD with a limited sex life if your partner has an infection.

In addition, some STDs can be harbored inside the body for years without a visible trace. That means a five-, ten-, or even fifteen-year monogamous relationship still does not ensure that you—or your partner—are disease-free.

HOT TUBS, HEALTH CLUBS, AND STDs

Although all STDs can be transmitted during sex, under certain conditions some can also be contracted in other ways. That is another reason why these bacteria and viruses have spread so rapidly. The most risky environments are these:

- ◆ Hot tubs   ◆ Steam rooms
- ◆ Saunas   ◆ Bathrooms
- ◆ The showers and dressing areas of some health clubs

Because their atmosphere is similar to the moist, warm conditions found in your genital area, these environments can make excellent breeding grounds for certain bacteria and viruses. In fact, touching your genital area with a contaminated towel can provide enough of a transmission factor to allow you to become infected. Because your body is often unprotected when you are using these facilities, your risk of infection via casual contact increases even further.

WHAT CAN YOU CATCH THROUGH CASUAL CONTACT?

Venereal warts, Gardnerella, yeast infections, and herpes can all be contracted nonsexually. Contact with active syphilis lesions or gonorrheal discharge could allow for nonsexual transmission as well.

HOW YOUR RISKS INCREASE

While having sex with an infected partner is the foremost way you can contract an STD, other factors will increase your risk as well:

- ◆ *A previous bout with an STD.* If you have had an STD in the past, studies show your chances for contracting one again are increased.
- ◆ *Age.* The younger woman, especially the teenager, is at a higher risk for STDs primarily because the uterus remains partially open until early to mid-twenties, allowing for easier passage of any number of bacteria into the body.
- ◆ *Choice of birth control.* Since one of the best forms of protection against STDs is provided by barrier methods of contraception, using a condom and/or a diaphragm can help decrease your risk of infection. Conversely, the pill offers no protection, and an IUD may actually increase your risk of infection by allowing for easier passage of bacteria into your system.

HOW STDs CAN AFFECT A WOMAN'S FERTILITY

Once an STD microorganism is allowed to pass from your vagina into your reproductive tract, an acute inflammation of your cervix (a condition called cervicitis) results. If left untreated, that infection can easily pass into your uterus and from there into your fallopian tubes and your ovaries. As these organs become infected, PID results. As you read in Chapter Two, depending on the organ involved, once PID occurs, your entire reproductive system may be placed in jeopardy.

HOW STDs CAN AFFECT A MAN'S FERTILITY

Because the bacteria and viruses associated with STDs first make contact with the male body via the penis, it is extremely easy for these microorganisms to enter a man's system. They do so by moving up through the urethra (the narrow shaft inside the penis), causing an infection called urethritis. Then, by working through the vas deferens (the hollow tubes that lead from the penis), they can attack the prostate gland, causing prostatitis. If they continue traveling to the epididymis (the small gland located on top of each testicle), an infection called epididymitis results. Finally, an STD can invade the testicle.

Infections that go on indefinitely without treatment can not only impair the organs themselves (resulting in defective or no sperm), but can also cause an abundance of scar tissue. This can result in serious blockages in the reproductive system that can inhibit both sperm maturity and travel.

Finally, if an STD invades the testicles, permanent sterility can result.

WHAT EVERY COUPLE CAN DO TO PROTECT FERTILITY: AN STD PRIMER

The most essential part of STD protection is the care you give yourself in the form of body awareness. To help you and your partner get a head start on the protection you *both* need, use the following STD primer to learn what to look for in each of your bodies, along with the fast, easy treatments that can help you avoid future problems.

GONORRHEA

Signs and Symptoms:

FEMALE BODY

♦ Mild genital burning and/or itching

- Slight vaginal discharge
- Frequent urge to urinate and/or urinary discomfort

MALE BODY

- Yellow, puslike penile discharge that rapidly increases in volume, and is much thicker than the normal mucous secretions of arousal.
- Penile discomfort (primarily at tip) two to five days after being infected
- Painful and/or burning urination

Potential Reproductive Damage: Most commonly affects fallopian tubes in women, constriction and closure of all sperm passageways in men.

Test: Since there are so many bacteria capable of being confused with those causing gonorrhea, a culture of vaginal fluids that allows only the growth of this microorganism is still the best method of detection for women. For men, a culture of the ejaculatory fluid is needed.

High-Risk Factors: Multiple partners, an infected partner.

Treatment: Broad-spectrum antibiotics, including tetracycline; an injectible drug, spectinomycin hydrochloride; and some penicillin-related drugs like ampicillin. In certain individuals an untreated infection may cure itself in anywhere from a few weeks (in men) to a year (in women). However, chances of reproductive and other bodily damage increase when no treatment is provided.

For Your Information:

- Gonorrhea can be spread to the eyes and lead to irreversible blindness.
- Oral sex with an infected partner can result in gonorrhea of the throat, the most common symptom of which is a sore throat. This form is less contagious.
- Condoms can dramatically cut the risk of infection and should always be used if the activities of your partner or his physical symptoms are in question.

Warning for Men: Two out of every ten men who contract gonorrhea do not have symptoms. They must rely on the honesty of their partner to inform them that they have been exposed. Any man who is told of gonorrheal contact should be tested and treated immediately, even if no symptoms are present.

In addition, often right after infection and sometimes before any symptoms appear, a slight irritation stimulates the nerve endings in the penis, causing a man to feel an increased desire for sex. This is one of the reasons the disease can be so easily spread.

CHLAMYDIA TRACHOMATIS INFECTION

Signs and Symptoms:

FEMALE BODY

- Slight discharge and some vaginal burning for the first three or four days after becoming infected.
- Very often, there are no signs or symptoms.

MALE BODY

- White discharge from penis
- Frequent urge to urinate and/or some burning

Potential Reproductive Damage:

- In some women, chlamydia infection can give rise to vaginal changes that create a hostile environment capable of damaging or killing sperm.
- It can affect the lining of the womb, leading to premature birth, still birth, or neonatal death.
- It may lead to salpingitis, an inflammation of the fallopian tubes.
- In men, chlamydia is the leading cause of nongonococcal urethritis (NGU), an infection that can attack the prostate gland and the epididymis. In severe cases it can cause so much scar tissue that complete infertility results.

Tests: There is a vaginal culture specifically for chlamydia. Men should get a semen culture.

High-Risk Factors: For women: IUD use, youth. For both sexes: multiple partners or an infected partner.

Treatment:

- Broad-spectrum antibiotics, such as tetracycline or doxycycline (Vibramycin), taken orally for seven to twenty days.
- Occasionally the body's own immune system can overpower the chlamydia microorganism and stop the infection on its own. This, however, is rare and should never be relied upon as a cure.

For Your Information:

- If you are sexually active, with multiple partners, or if the activities of your current partner are in question, you should have a chlamydia test every six months.
- Tests for chlamydia are not 100 percent accurate, especially if the disease has progressed from your cervix into your fallopian tubes. For this reason, always seek treatment if your sex partner is diagnosed as having this disease.
- Use of a contraceptive sponge and/or condoms containing the spermicide nonoxynol-9 during sex can offer an extra measure of protection against transmission of the chlamydia bacteria.

CONDYLOMA ACUMINATA (VENEREAL WARTS)

Signs and Symptoms:

FEMALE BODY

- Firm dark pink or red growths that usually appear in clusters on the vulva, or outer vagina. In some women these growths cause itching, irritation, or bleeding.
- Warts can also appear on the side walls of the vagina or even on the cervix itself, in which case they can be seen only during a gyn exam.
- Warts can spread from the vagina into the anal area on their own, without anal sex.

MALE BODY

- Warts may appear on the penis or anywhere in the genital area.
- Warts may also appear in the anal region if transmission took place in a homosexual encounter, or if this area of a male's body came in contact with a toilet seat, towel, or any moist, warm environment in which the virus was living.

Potential Reproductive Damage:

- Caused by one strain of the powerful human papilloma virus (HPV), genital warts can be a forerunner to cervical abnormalities, some of which have been implicated in the development of cervical cancer.
- Venereal warts in the vagina may contribute to a hostile environment, inhibiting or disrupting conception.
- Since pregnancy stimulates the development of almost any growth, venereal warts present after conception can grow so large that they can block the vagina and/or the birth canal and increase the risk of cesarean delivery.
- The potential for reproductive damage in men is not completely known.

Tests: For women: the ViraPap and the traditional Pap smear. For men: on-site inspection of genitals.

High-Risk Factors:

- Youth: Young women in their teens and early twenties are at highest risk, especially if they have more than one sexual partner.
- Smoking
- Birth control pills
- History of genital herpes

Treatment:

- Removal of warts with an application of podophylin, an acid that chemically "burns" away the virus. Your doctor must apply the treatment to each wart individually, and several repeat treatments may be necessary for complete cure.
- If warts do not respond to treatment with podophylin, they can be treated via electrocauterization, which helps burn the warts and destroys the virus.
- While laser surgery has been used to treat warts, there have recently been some setbacks with this method. Tests made under the guidance of Dr. Jerome M. Garden of Northwestern University Medical School in Chicago showed this treatment may cause the virus to spread to other parts of the body, as well as to those present in the operating environment, via the smoke that is emitted during the vaporization process. The virus has, for example, been found on the vocal cords of operating room personnel.
- Other treatments include freezing the warts with liquid nitrogen and

injections directly into the affected area three times weekly with an antiviral drug, interferon alpha-2B (Intron A).

For Your Information

- ◆ Since venereal warts can be transmitted via casual contact as well as sexually, remain acutely aware of any symptoms and/or be tested immediately if signs of this disease appear.
- ◆ Since moist, warm towels, public showers, saunas, and steam rooms make excellent breeding grounds for this virus, be tested regularly with the new ViraPap smear if you normally find yourself in these environments.
- ◆ Because this disease is highly contagious, regular testing is advised if your partner or any close family member has been diagnosed as having venereal warts.

T-MYCOPLASMA INFECTION

Signs and Symptoms:
Male and female body: generally none, although some individuals may experience a slight burning during urination and a light, odorless discharge.

High-Risk Factors: Multiple partners.

Tests: A vaginal culture or a sperm check for the specific T-mycoplasma bacterium.

Treatment: Ampicillin or tetracycline taken orally for seven to fourteen days, or other antibiotics, depending on culture sensitivity.

Potential Reproductive Damage:

- ◆ Although no link has been found between the T-mycoplasma organism and infertility (it does not, for example, cause PID), when the organism is present in either the male or the female body at the time of conception, there may be an increased risk of miscarriage.
- ◆ In men, T-mycoplasma is responsible for up to 25 percent of all occurrences of nongonococcal urethritis.

For Your Information:

- T-mycoplasma is still a relatively new disease, discovered in Europe in the 1970s and found in significant numbers in the United States only since the early 1980s. For this reason, information about the microorganism itself and any potential damage it can cause is still largely inconclusive. It has been verified as playing an important role in miscarriage, however, often upping the risk factor by a significant margin. Since recent evidence shows that a man who harbors T-mycoplasma bacteria may contribute to his wife's increased risk of miscarriage, if you are having repeated difficulty carrying to term, you and your partner should both be checked for the presence of this disease.
- Because this disease is usually totally silent, the occurrence of even one miscarriage should be grounds to request a culture, especially if you have never been tested.

SYPHILIS

Signs and Symptoms (General—Male and Female Body)

FIRST SIGN: CHANCRE

- The chancre (pronounced "shanker") is a sore that appears anywhere from two weeks to two months following initial contact with an infected partner.
- It is usually brownish in color, hard in texture, and often resembles a large pimple. There can be one chancre or a cluster, and they are usually painless.
- Chancres can appear almost anywhere on the body where contact has been made with the infection: fingers, mouth, breasts, rectum. Most often they occur in the genital area. In women they can be internal and/or hidden in the folds of the vagina.
- While chancres are the usual sign, they don't appear in every case, and they usually disappear on their own, even when not treated. The disease, however, remains in the body and produces what is called secondary syphilis.

SECONDARY SYPHILIS

- From a few weeks to a few months after the chancre disappears, a brownish rash resembling German measles may result. The most

common sites are the palms of hands, soles of feet, mouth, and nose.
◆ There are flulike symptoms, swollen lymph nodes, and fatigue, lasting about two weeks.
◆ Untreated, these symptoms disappear, and the disease seems to be gone, sometimes for many years. The microorganism responsible for syphilis lives on, however, continuously multiplying in your body. In time it causes extensive damage, including heart disease, paralysis, insanity, blindness, and eventually death.

Potential Reproductive Damage:

◆ During the "silent" period, the years when no symptoms are present, the disease can easily be passed on to any fetus that is conceived, any baby born to a mother who is infected.
◆ If syphilis is active during the first trimester of pregnancy, there is also an increased risk of miscarriage, premature labor and congenital malformations.
◆ In men the syphilis virus causes no direct, specific reproductive damage. However, by contaminating his partner, a man with syphilis can indirectly cause severe damage to the pregnancy.

High-Risk Factors: Sex with an infected partner, multiple partners.

Tests:

◆ *Early stages.* The "darkfield examination," a method of examining the chancres through a microscope for an on-site diagnosis.
◆ *Later stages.* There are three basic blood tests:
    Venereal disease research laboratory (VDRL) test
    Fluorescent treponema antibodies (FTA) absorption test
    Rapid plasma reagin (RPR) test

The VDRL and RPR are fast, inexpensive, and easy, but they can show a "false positive," indicating syphilis where none exists. The FTA is more accurate but generally takes longer and can be more expensive to perform.

Treatment:

◆ An injection of long-acting penicillin
◆ In advanced or stubborn cases, a second or even third injection may be needed at one-week intervals.

For Your Information:

- While relegated to a medical backseat for quite a number of years, syphilis has been making a comeback of late, with an alarming number of new cases developing each year. For this reason, don't assume this disease belongs to another generation.
- Because it can attack any tissue or organ of the body, it often causes destruction throughout your entire system. It is not only a painful disease, but a deadly one that you cannot afford to dismiss.

GENITAL HERPES

Signs and Symptoms:

FEMALE BODY

- Clusters of small blisters on a reddened area of skin that eventually break and form small scabs and sores. They can be painful and usually itch.
- Most often they appear in and around the outside of the vagina, the most common site being the labia, or outer lips.
- Signs and symptoms appear anywhere from two to ten days after contact with the disease.
- *Initial outbreak.* There are swollen glands, particularly in the groin, with a slight fever and flulike symptoms.
- *Prior to any outbreak.* The vagina may be red and feel sore, swollen, and itchy.

MALE BODY

- Same as in the female body, with lesions appearing mostly on the tip or the shaft of the penis.

Potential Reproductive Damage:

- An active herpes infection at the time of delivery can cause your newborn to contract the disease. Since infants have little or no immunity to infection, the virus can literally ravage their tiny, defenseless bodies.
- As many as 25 percent of all newborns who contract herpes die. If the virus attacks their eyes, they can be permanently blinded.

◆ In men a herpes infection can cause nongonococcal urethritis (NGU) in up to 10 percent of all cases.

High-Risk Factors: Sex with an infected partner, lowered immune system due to stress, illness or fatigue.

Test: Diagnosis is made on sight by a qualified professional.

Treatment:

◆ Acyclovir, a medication offered in both internal and external forms, has been shown to provide some *relief* of symptoms and to decrease the length of an episode.
◆ Since no antibiotic has been found to be effective in treating viruses, there is no cure for herpes.

For Your Information:

◆ Once in your system, the herpes virus continues to reactivate at intervals, the length of time between outbreaks varying for each individual.
◆ Herpes cannot be spread during a remission period. However, there is evidence that once the virus becomes active in the body (as it does several days prior to the appearance of symptoms), it can be transmitted.
◆ Because at certain stages herpes lesions can resemble syphilis, it's important that all cases be verified by a physician as soon as symptoms appear.
◆ Herpes outbreaks may be exacerbated by stress, which lowers the functioning of the immune system and allows the virus to go from its dormant state to an active one.
◆ No related diseases (including herpes simplex, which causes cold sores; herpes zoster, which causes shingles; chickenpox; Epstein–Barr syndrome; or cytomegalovirus) provide an immunity against genital herpes.

VAGINITIS

While many forms of vaginitis can be self-generated (that is, they develop within the body, without the invasion of any outside bacteria or viruses), they are generally not communicable. However, there *are* three types that can be sexually transmitted and are found both in the male and in the female body:

- Candidiasis (yeast infection)
- Trichomoniasis
- Gardnerella infection

For this reason many doctors choose to categorize them as STDs.

YEAST INFECTIONS

Medically termed moniliasis or candidiasis, a yeast infection results when the delicate alkaline–acid balance of the mouth, vagina, or rectum is biochemically disrupted, allowing the healthy flora that normally live in these areas to start growing out of control. The result is a fungus infection that can spread rapidly throughout the body. When the genitals are involved, this infection can be transmitted during sexual activity.

High-Risk Factors:

- Stress
- Antibiotics
- Sex with an infected partner
- Allergies
- Hormone imbalance

Signs and Symptoms:

A chronic yeast infection can cause a variety of diseases and conditions:

- Depression
- Diarrhea
- Migraine headaches
- Anxiety
- Constipation
- PMS
- Bloating
- Acne
- Joint pain

For this reason, signs and symptoms of a yeast infection can take almost any form and appear anywhere in the body. However, when it develops as a result of sexual contact, the first signs and symptoms are usually concentrated in the genital tract.

FEMALE BODY

- Discharge (thick and white, similar to cottage cheese, with a "yeasty" odor)
- Itching
- Burning (particularly on the labia, or lips of the vagina)
- Sometimes painful intercourse
- Reddening of the vagina, the irritation and subsequent pain spreading into your rectum, making sitting or even walking very painful

MALE BODY

- ◆ Genital itching
- ◆ Genital rash
- ◆ Penile discharge

Potential Reproductive Damage:

- ◆ A yeast infection in the vagina may interfere with sperm transport, hampering sperm's ability to reach your egg.
- ◆ It can also increase the acid level in the vagina, making it difficult for sperm to survive.
- ◆ In men, yeast infections can cause an inflammation of both the urethra and the prostate gland and thus affect sperm transport. There is also some evidence that the yeast fungus can attach to sperm, weighing it down and causing motility problems.

Treatment: Current treatment for yeast infections in women include antifungal suppositories and creams like:

- ◆ Nystatin
- ◆ Monistat
- ◆ Femstat

For men, Nystatin taken orally in tablet or powder form is most often prescribed.

In addition, diet modification has been shown to have a positive effect on rebalancing the normal floral levels and eliminating the yeast fungus both in men and in women.

FOODS THAT MAY INHIBIT A YEAST INFECTION

- ◆ Yogurt
- ◆ Cranberry juice
- ◆ Garlic

FOODS TO AVOID

- ◆ All yeast products
- ◆ Refined sugars and carbohydrates
- ◆ Fermented foods (including miso soup, soy sauce, vinegar)
- ◆ Dried fruits
- ◆ Peanuts (dry roasted)

For Your Information:

While monilial infections in the mouth are usually caused by antibiotic medication, they can also be transmitted via oral sex. When this occurs, the mouth becomes red and inflamed with cheesy white patches that bleed when scraped.

TRICHOMONIASIS

The microorganism responsible for the condition known as trichomoniasis (*Trichomonas vaginalis*) is a parasite that can live in the vagina and, in the male, in the urethra or prostate gland, and is passed on during sexual intercourse. Capable of causing a chronic infection that is often symptomless, it can live silently inside the body for many years. When it is finally activated (due to changes in the genital environment brought about by stress or other illnesses, for example), it is often difficult or even impossible to ascertain when or from whom you contracted this parasite.

Signs and Symptoms:

Once this parasite becomes active in a woman's body, the following symptoms can appear:

- Yellow-green vaginal discharge
- Foul vaginal odor
- Severe itching
- Irritated genital membranes
- Painful urination
- Painful intercourse

Should the infection spread to the uterus, pelvic pain can also result.

In the man's body the primary symptom is a yellow-green penile discharge and genital itching.

Potential Reproductive Damage:

While studies linking trichomoniasis and reproductive health are still inconclusive, I believe that because this parasite is associated with changes in the vaginal environment, it can contribute to conception difficulties and/or increase the risk of miscarriage. In men it may interfere with fertility by attaching to sperm and affecting transport. Once diagnosed and treated, however, trichomoniasis should have no residual effects on your ability to conceive.

Treatment:

- The standard treatment in women is a 250-milligram tablet of metronidazole (Flagyl) taken orally three times a day; this usually brings about a full cure in about ten days. Alternative treatment can include a megadose of two grams of metronidazole taken in twenty-four hours.

- ◆ In men the general treatment is 250 milligrams of metronidazole taken twice daily for ten days or one megadose of two grams taken in twenty-four hours.
- ◆ Intercourse should be avoided during treatment, and both partners must be treated simultaneously (even if only one of you has symptoms) in order to avoid reinfection.

Warning: The Misdiagnosis You Must Avoid

The most accurate diagnostic measure for detecting trichomoniasis in women is a Pap smear and/or a direct examination of the discharge itself under a microscope; the latter is also the method used to detect this condition in men. Some doctors believe correct diagnosis can be made after a pelvic exam alone, but I must caution you against this. I have often seen monilial infections mistaken for trichomoniasis and consequently mistreated with metronidazole. Since that medication can exacerbate monilial symptoms and actually worsen this infection, treatment for trichomoniasis should never be accepted without proper documentation that the disease does indeed exist in your system.

GARDNERELLA INFECTION

One of the most common forms of vaginitis is caused by *Gardnerella vaginalis;* it can be transmitted on clothing or towels and is considered highly contagious. However, it is most often passed on during sexual intercourse. Because the gardnerella bacterium can hide so comfortably in a man's body, often showing few if any symptoms, it can be transmitted silently. Once inside *your* body it can be equally elusive and thus hard to diagnose.

Signs and Symptoms:

- ◆ The only female symptom produced by this bacteria is a grayish-white discharge with an extremely unpleasant odor.
- ◆ It does *not* cause any local irritation, swelling or itching.
- ◆ In men the only symptom is a penile discharge. Often there are no symptoms.

Potential Reproductive Damage:

Although gardnerella exists in your reproductive system, curiously enough it causes no harm to your organs, no matter how long it resides in your body. However, its presence can create a hostile vaginal environment and so alter the ability of your partner's sperm to reach or fertilize your egg.

In men, gardnerella can lead to infections of the reproductive glands, affecting both the organs themselves and the quality of the sperm produced.

Warning: Increased Risk of Miscarriage

Should conception occur while a woman is harboring a gardnerella infection, her chances for miscarriage increase. For this reason many doctors now routinely prescribe certain antibiotics, namely, erythromycin or penicillin, for any woman who gets pregnant and has a repeated history of miscarriage.

Diagnosis and Treatment:

Gardnerella is diagnosed by taking a sample of your vaginal secretions or of your partner's sperm and examining it under a microscope for the presence of certain clue cells. Although these cells can sometimes be present when no gardnerella infection exists, adding a drop of potassium hydroxide to the slide will, when the disease is present, cause a strong fishy odor.

The treatment of gardnerella is often determined by the sensitivity of the culture, but antibiotics like tetracycline, ampicillin, and cephalexin (Keflex) are often prescribed for seven to ten days.

AIDS

Acquired immune deficiency syndrome (AIDS) is, of course, the most deadly of all STDs. Since there is currently no cure and it appears that all who contract AIDS eventually die of the disease, it seems almost pointless, even cruel, to discuss it in the same breath as fertility. However, since an AIDS diagnosis can be elusive for up to ten years, it's possible that a woman who unknowingly has the disease could conceive during that time.

A Warning: AIDS and Your Unborn Baby!

Fifty percent of all babies born to mothers with AIDS or conceived by fathers or mothers who have the disease contract the AIDS virus as well. AIDS is a nondiscriminating killer. It attacks adults, children, and newborn babies of either sex, and being married or in a monogamous relationship does not guarantee immunity.

STDs: ARE YOU AT RISK?

To help round out your knowledge not only of STDs, but of the ways in which they can affect your life, here are some of the most commonly asked questions about these diseases, along with the answers that can help you relax and enjoy your sexuality for years to come.

Q: Can I get an STD from kissing?

A: Generally, no. However, since gonorrhea is capable of living in the throat, it may possibly be transmitted this way. In addition, any open sores in your mouth, such as fever blisters or dental lesions, could up your chances of infection of oral gonorrhea.

While the AIDS virus is not generally transmitted via saliva, there are still some conflicting reports as to the role that deep mouth kissing may play in transmitting *this* disease.

Q: I had PID in the past. Does this mean I won't ever get pregnant?

A: No. It is the extent and severity of your PID, and whether you were treated promptly, that determine whether your fertility was affected. If no scar tissue formed and there was no damage to your fallopian tubes, your chances of achieving a natural conception are good. In addition, even if damage has been done, a laser laparoscopy or some form of microsurgery could help reverse any problems that did occur, allowing you to conceive.

If, however, your tubes underwent severe damage, you might need some laboratory assistance, such as in vitro fertilization, to help you get pregnant. (Review the discussion of PID and its link to infertility in Chapter Two, pages 18–21.)

Q: My husband and I both had gonorrhea in college and were treated with penicillin. Could we be sterile now?

A: Most likely not, if you were treated immediately and PID was not diagnosed.

Q: Can I get an STD from oral sex?

A: Yes. During oral sex, gonorrhea, herpes, syphilis, yeast infections, and possibly AIDS (if an open sore in the mouth is present), as well as a few lesser-known STDs, *can* be transmitted. If sores appear in your mouth or a sore throat develops a few days after oral sex, report these symptoms to your doctor and request cultures and tests for these diseases.

Q: Is it true you can't get an STD from just one encounter?

A: No. You can catch an STD any time you have sex with an infected partner. Your chances for catching any disease increase the more times you are exposed, but you are at great risk even after one encounter with a person carrying an STD.

Q: Can I have an STD and not know it?

A: Yes. Chlamydia, venereal warts, T-mycoplasma and gonorrhea can all be symptom-free or have signs that appear only for a short period of time and then disappear. Just because the symptoms are gone, however, doesn't mean the disease has been cured. Chlamydia can linger for years, with a slow, silent means of destroying your organs, while gonorrhea can wreak havoc in the few days before symptoms become apparent.

Q: Can an STD disappear by itself:

A: Yes. Several, like gonorrhea, can burn out on their own, after causing destruction. Syphilis can also disappear for ten or twenty years and then reappear. In addition, there is evidence that venereal warts disappear on their own. However, since it is almost impossible for you to tell if a disease has disappeared or is merely "hiding" silently in your body, never take a lack of symptoms as a sign that all is well. Be cultured and tested any and every time a possibility for infection exists, and begin treatment immediately if any of these diseases are discovered in your body.

Q: I was a virgin when I got married and never slept with any man but my husband. Could I get an STD?

A: Yes. If your husband was sexually active before marriage, he could have been harboring a silent infection in his prostate gland that was ultimately passed on to you. The most common are T-mycoplasma, chlamydia, gardnerella, and venereal warts.

Q: Can an STD get into my reproductive system during anal sex?

A: Not directly, although many bacteria that are deposited in the rectum during anal sex can work their way into the vagina later on and then penetrate your pelvic region. Chances of this increase during exceptionally vigorous vaginal penetration, which can drive any bacteria or viruses present in your vagina deeper into your system. Your partner *must* cleanse his penis thoroughly before attempting vaginal sex after anal penetration.

You can also increase your risks via improper wiping and/or cleansing after a bowel movement. To help protect yourself, always wipe front to back, away from the vagina.

Q: I just found out my husband has an STD. Does this mean he had sex outside our marriage?

A: It could, of course, mean that. However, it could also mean he was harboring the disease in his body long before he met you—or that his infection came from an infection you may be unknowingly harboring in *your* body. In addition, since some STDs are spread nonsexually as well as through intercourse, it's possible your husband contracted his disease in a totally innocent encounter with a wet towel or unsanitary sauna or steam room.

Q: Can I get an STD from a toilet?

A: Yes, but not all STDs are equally contagious in this manner. Some bacteria and viruses, such as those responsible for herpes, yeast infections, and venereal warts, live outside the body longer than others, so transmission via toilet seats, vibrators, or any other object that comes in contact with your genital area can more easily occur. Other microorganisms, such as chlamydia, T-mycoplasma, and those causing gonorrhea, usually don't live outside the body very long, so your genitals would have to come in contact with an object, say, a toilet seat, almost immediately after vaginal or penile fluids of an infected person had been deposited. While this time factor significantly reduces the risk of transmitting many STDs in this manner, transmission can still happen. To be safe, always use a paper toilet seat cover when using any public facility or the bathroom of any person you suspect may be infected.

A FINAL WORD: SAFE SEX, NOT FEARFUL SEX

While the perils of a sexually active life cannot be denied, this chapter was not meant to scare or inhibit you or to decrease your ability to enjoy sex in any way. It was written to help you demystify some of the physical problems that can arise in the course of a sexual relationship and help you keep those problems from affecting your health and your fertility, now and in the future.

It was also meant to help you understand your own body better and thus spot trouble signs before the problem arises. My intention has been to reassure you that, whatever the ways you have enjoyed sex in the past or will enjoy it in the future, you can protect yourself from *any* and *all* problems.

· 5 ·

YOUR FERTILITY FROM NINE TO FIVE

The Reproductive Hazards of the Workplace—and How Every Couple Can Avoid Them

Mary Ellen lay quietly in her bed, her hands resting atop her now-protruding tummy. Five months pregnant and just beginning to feel life, she senses a rush of anxiety each time her baby moves inside her. Although she is healthy and strong (and a sonogram shows her baby is fine as well), Mary Ellen lives in constant fear of miscarriage. Why? She just found out that seven out of every ten women in her office complex have miscarried in the past eight months. The health department is looking into the matter, but by the time any answers arrive, Mary Ellen's fate—and that of her unborn baby—will already have been decided.

"If only I had known what was going on," she told me, "I would have quit my job before trying to get pregnant."

THE WORKPLACE AND YOUR FERTILITY

Astonishingly, recent studies show that reproductive disorders are among the top ten work-related illnesses for *both sexes*. Currently, there are more than 14 million *men and women* exposed to potential reproductive hazards on the job every day. In fact, a recent report by the

75

U.S. Office of Technology Assessment revealed that out of the sixty thousand chemicals currently in widespread use in United States industry, only three are regulated in part on consideration of human reproductive health. In short, no matter what you do for a living, the workplace and its potential for affecting both male and female fertility is now a major issue—and one that no couple in their childbearing years can afford to ignore.

REPRODUCTIVE HAZARDS: WHO IS AT RISK

Because each workplace has its own specific hazards, it's often difficult to generalize the risk factors. However, when problems do occur they are usually linked to one of the following factors:

- Exposure to radiation, including that from copy machines, computer terminals, and fax machines
- Contaminated and/or low-oxygenated air due to poor ventilation, dirty heating or air-conditioning systems, or chemical pollutants
- Direct contact with toxic chemicals, including those used for copy machines and printing devices, as well as those used in various manufacturing processes
- Dangerously high temperatures—especially hazardous for male fertility
- Atmospheric pressure, which can contribute to premature labor or miscarriage

These factors could be present in the specific job tasks that you or your mate perform, or they could be fundamental to the nature of your company's business, including what it manufactures, processes, ships, or stores. Moreover, toxic elements not used by you but by others in your workplace could harm you by polluting the general atmosphere.

Depending on the substance or substances, how long you have been exposed, and, most important, the level to which you are exposed on a regular basis, a variety of reproductive problems can occur:

- Fertilization difficulties
- Implantation problems
- Ovulation interference
- Menstrual irregularities
- Increased risk of miscarriage
- Increased risk of birth defects
- Decrease in libido (sex drive)

In addition, there can be problems even after your baby is born. Studies show that contaminants to which you are exposed on a regular basis can show up in your breast milk, making breast-feeding a potential hazard that could result in an increased risk of cancer, respiratory problems, or immune system deficiencies for your baby.

YOU AND YOUR PARTNER—AT EQUAL RISK

Although much of the attention on the workplace–fertility link has been in regard to women, the problems are by no means limited to the female population. A man's fertility can be so vulnerable to some workplace hazards that his reproductive system can experience damage in less time and with less exposure than a woman's. Making matters worse, many exployers continue to ignore male reproductive hazards. According to a new study conducted by the Massachusetts Occupational Health Program:

- ◆ Out of the 198 chemical and electronic firms queried on reproductive hazards, *only one* took the importance of male fertility into consideration by restricting hazardous jobs for those men whose partners were trying to conceive.
- ◆ Fewer than half the companies surveyed provided workers with any information about the reproductive risks of their jobs.

How can reproductive hazards threaten your mate's fertility? When exposed to certain harmful factors, he can experience one or more of the following problems on a temporary or even a long-term basis:

- ◆ Lowered sperm count
- ◆ Higher rate of abnormal sperm
- ◆ Increased risk of birth defects
- ◆ Sperm motility defects
- ◆ Testicle damage
- ◆ Impotence
- ◆ Loss of sex drive

In addition, the effects on him can also increase *your* risk of miscarriage.

THE GOOD NEWS: THE WORKPLACE CAN BE A SAFE PLACE!

The good news is that there are many ways your workplace can be made safer, for general good health and to protect your fertility. Laws have already been passed to ensure valuable reproductive rights; you'll read about them in this chapter. In addition, you and your partner can both take steps to eliminate work-related fertility hazards. A good place to start is by identifying the potential problems.

COMPUTERS AND YOUR FERTILITY: WHAT YOU NEED TO KNOW RIGHT NOW

Because much of what has been alleged about computers and infertility is based on rumor rather than fact, it is likely that some of what you have heard on this subject is untrue. However, important new information *has* recently surfaced indicating a link between computer use and specific, fertility-related problems, including:

◆ Increased risk of miscarriage
◆ Increased risk of birth defects
◆ Decreased fertility overall for men and women

For a long time most of these problems seemed to appear in *clusters:* isolated groups of computer workers in various industries in different geographic locations reported increases in reproductive problems, particularly miscarriages and birth defects. Because, however, the effects were not universal, many skeptics doubted the existence of this high-tech infertility. Recently, however, a study of over 1,500 women conducted by the Kaiser-Permanente Medical Group in northern California exploded the cluster theory, showing that computer-related fertility consequences are much more broadly based than anyone had realized. After following the pregnancies of 1,583 women, it was learned that

◆ Those who spent more than twenty hours per week working at a video display terminal (VDT) had twice as many miscarriages in the first three months of their pregnancy as did workers who did not use computers.
◆ When compared to nonusers, women who were exposed to just five hours per day of VDT use had a 40 percent increase in the number of babies born with congenital malformations.

Whether problems result from exposure *before* or *after* conception is still not known, but the dangers posed by computers are obviously clear.

HOW COMPUTERS CAN HARM YOUR FERTILITY

According to the most recent research, the link between computers and reproductive problems is not the machine itself, but the VDT used to visualize the information. Most emit one or both of the following types of radiation:

◆ Extra-low frequency (ELF)
◆ Very low frequency (VLF)

Some experts report that exposure to either of these types of radiation can cause damage to various areas of the reproductive system, as well as to a developing fetus. The end result can be miscarriage, birth defects, or difficulty in conceiving. In addition, the effects of low-level radiation are thought to be synergistic—made worse by outside factors, such as medication you may be taking or chemicals in your work environment—so even minimal exposure can sometimes cause problems.

VDTs and Your Menstrual Cycle

A brand-new study by the School of Management at UMIST (University of Manchester, Institute of Science and Technology in Manchester, England) finds that prolonged exposure to the VLF radiation of VDTs can also bring about menstrual irregularities, including:

- Cramps
- Anxiety
- Irritability
- Stress
- Amenorrhea (loss of menstrual cycle)

This may prove to be another link to infertility.

Other studies have reported that continued exposure to either VLF or ELF radiation can cause a biological stress that manifests itself in improper brain metabolism and malfunctioning of the endocrine system, which produces the hormones responsible for reproduction. I believe this finding may provide another connection between menstrual problems, VDTs, and infertility.

VDTs and Male Fertility

Although much of the focus of VDT damage has been on female fertility, men are by no means immune to its effect. In fact, a man's reproductive system is *more* sensitive than yours to the effects of all radiation, and when exposed to even minimal levels, he can experience

- Decreased sperm count
- Testicle damage
- Hormonal upsets
- Chromosome damage within the sperm, leading to birth defects and miscarriage

Because the effects of radiation are cumulative, simply spending time in an environment where many VDTs are regularly used can take its toll on his reproductive health—and on the health of your baby.

WORKING ON COMPUTERS: THE GOOD NEWS

Whether your job entails regular, daily work at a computer terminal or just occasional exposure and/or use, there *are* things you can do to help reduce the reproductive hazards:

- Several companies are now manufacturing accessories to help cut exposure to VDT radiation, including shielded cables, specially designed work stations, and portable radiation monitors to measure important leakage.
- Safe Monitor™, a reportedly radiation-free display terminal, is believed able to remove the threat of radiation-related dangers in computer work. Manufactured by The Safe Company Inc. in Needham, Massachusetts, this new monitor substitutes a liquid-crystal display, the kind used in wristwatches and clock-radios, for the traditional radiation-emitting cathode ray tube display system. For extra safety, the monitor itself and all cables are shielded, making it the only reportedly 100 percent radiation-free monitor available. It is completely compatible with all IBM machines, and it works on home and office systems alike.
- Finally, there are steps you can take to minimize any harmful effects of the computer equipment you are working on right now—at home or in your office. 9 to 5—the National Organization of Working Women—has done a tremendous job in helping to research the VDT—infertility link and in educating women and men about computer safety. The following is a sample of its guidelines for making your computer safer for you and your baby:

How to Protect Your Fertility

- Since one source of VLF radiation is the flyback transformer located at the back of your monitor, stay clear of this area when doing other work tasks.
- Push the screen as far back as your work station will allow, so long as you can read it without straining. Most VDT radiation projects only about ten feet from the front or back of the monitor.
- Avoid doing noncomputer tasks or taking breaks near the side of your terminal, or turn the terminal off if you do.
- Arrange your office so that you are not sitting close to the back or the side of a coworker's terminal.
- Try to use a laptop or portable computer whenever possible, especially if you are pregnant. These machines eliminate some types of radiation and cut down on others.
- Avoid color monitors. The radiation is three to four times greater than that from a monochrome monitor.

◆ Insist that your employer provide periodic, thorough testing of VDTs for excessive radiation leaks, as well as regular maintenance to prevent problems from occurring. Systematic testing can prevent x-ray emissions due to design flaws or a malfunction in your system.

CAN A LEAD APRON PROTECT YOUR BABY?

Because a lead apron can shield one from the harmful effects of *some* radiation, many of my patients ask whether it can also protect against the harmful effects of VDTs. It cannot. A lead shield protects one *only* from the effects of ionizing radiation, which is negligible in VDTs. It offers no protection against nonionizing VLF or ELF radiation, which are thought to be the most significant sources of VDT-related fertility damage.

Moreover, continual, long-term use of a lead apron when you are pregnant adds a weight on your stomach that may be more harmful to your baby than any radiation.

ANOTHER IMPORTANT WARNING!

Don't be fooled by clever packaging or by unsubstantiated advertising claims about screens, monitors, and other computer accessories. A random sampling found that many "radiation-reduced" and "radiation-free" products only reduced one type of frequency, leaving the others barely changed or untouched. To be sure that the product you purchase gives you all the protection it advertises, write to the manufacturer for specifics—if possible, for *written* guarantees about the type and amount of radiation reduction provided.

THE WORKPLACE FERTILITY PROTECTION GUIDE

Although computer use may have the most potentially widespread effects on fertility, many other occupations can present reproductive risks. The following guide should help you determine if your job might be harming your fertility. Although every attempt has been made to provide the most accurate, up-to-date information, please note this guide is by no means complete.

◆ Some substances that test as safe today may prove to be hazardous later.
◆ Some things that are suspect today may be proved safe when further studies have been made.
◆ Some factors medical science simply has not explored, and just

because a substance doesn't appear in this—or any—guide does not automatically mean it's safe.

This guide also does not suggest that everyone who works at these jobs or in these industries is exposed to these substances, nor does it imply that everyone who is exposed is in definite danger. It simply represents guidelines to help you investigate the limitations your work might place on your ability to conceive and deliver a healthy baby, now or in the future. Occupations are listed alphabetically. Their order suggests no ranking as to danger or intensity of harm. The numbers in each list of potential damage refer back to the corresponding numbered item indicated as a potential hazard.

ARTIST (Fine)

Potential Hazard:
1. Manganese dioxide
2. Formaldehyde
3. Glycol ethers
4. Lead

Potential Damage:
Male:
1. Impotence, reduced sex drive, decreased fertility
2. No data available
3. Abnormal or reduced sperm count, decreased fertility
4. Impotence, reduced sex drive, abnormal or reduced sperm count, decreased fertility, miscarriage in wife

Female:
1. No data available
2. Menstrual irregularities
3. Increased risk of birth defects
4. Menstrual irregularities, decreased fertility, increased risk of miscarriage, birth defects, stillbirths, infant mortality, contaminated breast milk

AIRLINE PERSONNEL (pilot, navigator, flight attendant)

Potential Hazard:
Overexposure to high-altitude radiation

Potential Damage:

Male:
Decreased sperm count, increased risk of birth defects, decreased fertility, impotence

Female:
Increased risk of miscarriage, premature labor, menstrual irregularities

BAKER

Potential Hazard:
Elevated temperatures

Potential Damage:
Male:
Reduced sperm count

Female:
No data available

CERAMICS WORKER, CRAFTS WORKER

Potential Hazard:
1. Lead
2. Glycol ethers
3. Manganese dioxide

Potential Damage:
Male:
1. Impotence, abnormal or decreased sperm, decreased fertility, miscarriage in wife
2. Abnormal or reduced sperm, decreased fertility
3. Impotence or reduced sex drive, decreased fertility

Female:
1. Menstrual irregularities, decreased fertility, increased risk of miscarriage, stillbirths, infant mortality, contaminated breast milk.
2. Increased risk of birth defects
3. No data available

CHEMICAL LABORATORY WORKER

Potential Hazard:
1. Carbon tetrachloride.
2. Benzene

Potential Damage:
Male:
1. Decreased fertility
2. No data available

Female:
1. No data available
2. Menstrual irregularities, increased risk of stillbirths, low-birthweight babies

COMPUTER PERSONNEL (programmer, keyboard operator, technician)

Potential Hazard:
Radiation

Potential Damage:
See the section on VDTs earlier in this chapter.

COSMETICS MANUFACTURER OR WORKER

Potential Hazard:
1. Mercury compounds
2. Formaldehyde
3. Nitrosamine
4. Estrogen

Potential Damage:
Male:
1. Impotence, reduced sex drive, reduced sperm count, increase in abnormal sperm, decreased fertility
2. No data available
3. Chromosomal abnormalities and/or mutations
4. Decreased fertility

Female:
1. Menstrual irregularities, increased risk of miscarriage, stillbirth, infant mortality, birth defects
2. Irregular menstrual cycles
3. Chromosomal abnormalities/mutations
4. Ovulation upsets, hormonal imbalances

CLOTHING OR TEXTILE WORKER

Potential Hazard:
1. Tris (flame retardant)
2. Formaldehyde

Potential Damage:
Male:
1. Decreased fertility
2. No data available

Female:
1. No data available
2. Irregular menstrual cycles

DENTAL CARE PERSONNEL (dentist, nurse, hygienist)

Potential Hazard:
1. Anesthetic gases, nitrous oxide
2. X-radiation
3. Mercury

Potential Danger:
Male:
1. Abnormal or reduced sperm, miscarriage in wife, decreased fertility
2. Abnormal or reduced sperm, decreased fertility, chromosomal or genetic damage
3. Impotence or reduced sex drive, low sperm count, increase in abnormal sperm, decreased fertility

Female:
1. Decreased fertility
2. Menstrual irregularities, decreased fertility, increased risk of birth defects, possible rise in number of miscarriages and stillbirths
3. Menstrual irregularities, increased risk of miscarriage, stillbirth, or infant mortality, birth defects

DES MANUFACTURERS AND WORKERS

Potential Hazard:
Diethylstilbestrol

Potential Damage:
Male:
Abnormal or reduced sperm, decreased fertility

Female:
Increased risk of birth defects, contaminated breast milk

DRY CLEANERS

Potential Hazard:
Carbon tetrachloride

Potential Damage:
Male:
Reduced fertility

Female:
No data available

EXTERMINATOR

Potential Hazard:
Pesticides (dibromochloropropane, kepone, DDT, DBCP carbaryl, DDVP, malathion)

Potential Damage:
Male:
Decreased sperm count, decreased fertility

Female:
Menstrual irregularities, decreased fertility, contaminated breast milk

FOUNDRY OR OVEN WORKERS

Potential Hazard:
Elevated temperatures

Potential Damage:
Male:
Reduced sperm count

Female:
No data available

FARM OR AGRICULTURAL WORKER

Potential Hazard:
1. Pesticides (see Exterminator)
2. Arsenic

Potential Damage:
Male:
1. Decreased sperm count, decreased fertility
2. Reduced sperm, decreased fertility

Female:
1. Menstrual irregularities, decreased fertility, contaminated breast milk
2. Increased risk of miscarriage, stillbirth, infant mortality, low-birth-weight babies, birth defects

HAIRDRESSER, COSMETOLOGIST, OR BARBER

Potential Hazard:
1. Lead in hair dyes
2. Hairspray resins (polyvinylpyrrolidone)
3. Nail polish solvents

Potential Damage:
Male:
1. Reduced fertility
2. Decreased fertility, increased risk of miscarriage in wife, impotence
3. Decreased fertility

Female:
1. Reduced fertility
2. Increased risk of miscarriage, stillbirth, infant mortality
3. Menstrual irregularities, decreased fertility

HAZARDOUS-WASTE DISPOSAL WORKER

Potential Hazard:
Lead, PBBs

Potential Damage:
Male:
Impotence or reduced sex drive, increase in abnormal sperm, reduced sperm count, decreased fertility, increased risk of miscarriage in wife

Female:
Menstrual irregularities, decreased fertility, increased risk of miscarriage, stillbirth, or infant mortality, contaminated breast milk

HEALTH CARE WORKER

Potential Hazard:
Ethylene oxide (disinfectant), x-radiation,

Potential Damage:
Male:
Decreased fertility

Female:
Increased risk of miscarriage and birth defects, decreased fertility

LAWYER, PARALEGAL, LEGAL SECRETARY

Potential Hazard:
Computers, electric office equipment, stress

Potential Damage:
Male:
Reduced sperm count, decreased fertility (see the section on VDTs earlier in this chapter)

Female:
Increased risk of miscarriage and birth defects, menstrual irregularities (see the section on VDTs)

MEDICAL PERSONNEL (doctor, nurse, aide, technician)

Potential Hazard:
1. Anesthetic gases, nitrous oxide
2. Anticancer drugs

Potential Damage:
Male:
1. Low sperm count, increase in abnormal sperm, increased risk of miscarriage in wife
2. Impotence, reduced sex drive, low sperm count, abnormal sperm, decreased fertility

Female:
1. Increased risk of miscarriage
2. Increased risk of miscarriage, contaminated breast milk

PESTICIDE WORKER, FARMERS

Potential Hazard:
Job-related chemicals

Potential Damage:
Male and female:
See Exterminator

HOUSE PAINTER

Potential Hazard:
1. Boron
2. Cadmium
3. PCBs
4. Formaldehyde
5. Aromatic hydrocarbons
6. Glycol ethers

Potential Damage:
Male:
1. Impotence, reduced sex drive, low sperm count, abnormal sperm
2. Impotence, abnormal or reduced sperm count, decreased fertility
3. No data available
4. No data available
5. Decreased fertility
6. Abnormal or reduced sperm, decreased fertility

Female:
1. Increased risk of miscarriage, stillbirth, infant mortality, birth defects
2. Menstrual irregularities, low-birthweight babies, contaminated breast milk
3. Menstrual irregularities
4. Decreased fertility
5. Increased risk of birth defects

PERFUME INDUSTRY

Potential Hazard:
Benzene, other organic solvents

Potential Damage:
Male:
No data available

Female:
Menstrual irregularities, increased risk of low-birthweight babies, infant mortality, birth defects

PHOTOGRAPHIC PROCESSOR

Potential Hazard:
1. Formaldehyde
2. Glycol ethers

Potential Damage:
Male:
1. No data available
2. Decreased fertility

Female:
1. Menstrual irregularities
2. Increased risk of birth defects

POLICE OFFICER

Potential Hazard:
Lead, stress

Potential Damage:
Male:
Impotence or decreased sex drive, abnormal or reduced sperm, decreased fertility, increased risk of miscarriage in wife

Female:
Menstrual irregularities, decreased fertility, increased risk of miscarriage and stillbirth, contaminated breast milk

PRINTER OR GRAPHICS DESIGNER

Potential Hazard:
Ethylene glycol PD

Potential Damage:
Male:
Testicular atrophy, decreased sperm count, increase in birth defects

Female:
Increased risk of birth defects

PVC MANUFACTURER OR PROCESSOR

Potential Hazard:
Vinyl chloride

Potential Damage:
Male:
Decreased fertility, increased risk of miscarriage in wife, possible impotence and reduced sex drive

Female:
Increased risk of miscarriage, stillbirth, and infant mortality

RADAR OPERATORS (including air crew member and transmitter operator)

Potential Hazard:
Microwaves

Potential Damage:
Male and Female:
Decreased fertility

RUBBER WORKER

Potential Hazard:
1. Chloroprene
2. Vinyl chloride

Potential Damage:
Male:
1. Impotence, reduced sex drive, low sperm count, abnormal sperm, increased risk of miscarriage in wife
2. See PVC Manufacturer or Processor

Female:
1. Menstrual irregularities
2. Increased risk of miscarriage, stillbirths, and infant mortality

STOCKBROKER

Potential Hazard:
Computer terminals, low-voltage appliances (fax machines, tote boards, etc.) stress, carbon monoxide (cigarette smoke)

Potential Damage:
See the discussion of VDTs earlier in this chapter.
Male:
Reduced sperm count, abnormal sperm

Female:
Menstrual irregularities, increased risk of miscarriage and birth defects

STORAGE BATTERY WORKER

Potential Hazard:
Cadmium

Potential Damage:
Male:
Impotence, reduced sex drive, low sperm count, increase in abnormal sperm, decreased fertility

Female:
Increased risk of miscarriage and stillbirth, decreased fertility

SMELTERS

Potential Hazard:
1. Cadmium
2. Nickel
3. Manganese

Potential Damage:
Male:
1. See Storage Battery Worker
2. Reduced fertility
3. Impotence, reduced sex drive, decreased fertility

Female:
1. See Storage Battery Workers.
2. No data available
3. No data available

SOIL TREATER

Potential Hazard:
Carbon disulfide

Potential Damage:
Male:
Impotence, abnormal or low sperm count, increased risk of miscarriage in wife

Female:
Menstrual irregularities, increased risk of miscarriage

UTILITY WORKER

Potential Hazard:
1. Epichlorodrin
2. Ethylene oxide
3. 1,3 Butadiene

Potential Damage:
Male:
Decreased fertility (all three)

Female:
1. No data available
2. Increased risk of miscarriage, birth defects
3. Decreased fertility, increased risk of miscarriage and birth defects

VISCOSE RAYON WORKER

Potential Hazard:
Carbon disulfide

Potential Damage:
Male:
Impotence, abnormal or low sperm count, increased risk of miscarriage in wife

Female:
Menstrual irregularities, increased risk of miscarriage

WELDER

Potential Hazard:
Manganese, nickel

Potential Damage:
Male:
Impotence or reduced sex drive, decreased fertility

Female:
No data available

X-RAY INSPECTOR, TECHNICIAN

Potential Hazard:
Ionizing radiation, microwaves

Potential Damage:
Male:
Abnormal or reduced sperm, decreased fertility

Female:
Menstrual irregularities, decreased fertility, increased risk of birth defects

THE CHEMICALS
THAT CAN AFFECT
YOUR PREGNANCY

A wide variety of toxic substances found in the workplace not only affect your ability to *get* pregnant but can harm your baby after conception occurs. If you are pregnant, take special precautions to avoid overexposure to these substances:

- Anesthetic gases
- Dibromochloropropane
- Ethylene oxide
- Lead
- Methyl mercury
- Organic solvents
- Vinyl chloride

HOW TO MAKE YOUR WORKPLACE
A SAFE PLACE

Regardless of what occupation or field you or your partner are currently in, according to the federal Hazard Communication Standard, it is your unquestionable right to obtain information about any health hazard of your working environment, including those that can threaten your unborn baby, without fear of employer retribution. In many cities all across the United States, the Occupational Health and Safety Administration (OSHA) and/or the National Institute for Occupational Safety and Health (NIOSH), both found in the government listings of your phone book, can be helpful in providing you with information about your employer's *obligations for protecting you.* Here are just some of the things your employer is required by federal law to tell you:

- The existence of any hazardous chemicals present in your work environment: all hazardous material must be clearly marked as such, with the name and address of the supplier.
- Complete health and safety information about any hazardous chemicals present in your work environment: this should include the product name, possible health effects, symptoms resulting from exposure, and handling procedures.
- Full information on precautions you must take in working with these substances, including required protective clothing and/or equipment, as well as on emergency treatment in case of accident.

◆ The results of any company studies, exposure records, or air monitoring that could affect the health and safety of workers.

YOU CAN MAKE A DIFFERENCE!

In addition to taking advantage of the federal and state regulations already in effect, don't overlook your power to help initiate even more laws in your behalf. Remember, some of the most important changes in labor standards and practices have been brought about by employees who took an active, even aggressive role in job safety.

For example, in 1977 a group of male workers at a California plant manufacturing the chemical DCPB discovered over lunchtime conversation that none had been able to father a child since they'd begun their jobs. A subsequent semen analysis showed a marked decrease in the sperm counts of the men working with this chemical, many of them so low that they were completely sterile. The workers joined forces and fought for important changes. What started as a casual lunchtime chat turned into a major issue that eventually led to the government's banning the manufacture of DCPB.

SEVEN STEPS TO A SAFER WORKPLACE

If you do believe your working environment may be a threat to your fertility, I strongly urge you to take some kind of action right away. The following guidelines for a safer workplace were recently issued by Nine To Five, the National Organization of Working Women, and the Southeast Michigan Coalition on Occupational Health and Safety (SEMCOSH). They can help you obtain a safer, healthier environment for everyone.

1. Share your reproductive health concerns with other workers. Discover how many female coworkers, as well as how many wives of male coworkers, are having problems conceiving or have been plagued with an unusual number of miscarriages, premature labor, or babies born with birth defects. This may shed light on whether your workplace is suspect.
2. Document any problems you can clearly identify and then organize an employee task force to investigate specifics. Share your discoveries with your coworkers and encourage them to do the same. Pooling information can help everyone determine where specific problems might lie.
3. Discuss your concerns with your employer. You cannot be fired, punished, or discriminated against for inquiring or complaining about health and safety concerns of your job.

4. Request copies of all company studies concerning reproductive or other health hazards of your workplace. Your employer is required by law to share with you any significant health or safety information about your job.

5. If you have reason to believe that the air in your workplace may be contaminated, request that air samples be taken. If your employer refuses, contact your local Coalition on Occupational Health and Safety (listed in your phone book under government agencies).

6. File grievances with your employer, and encourage coworkers to do the same. If possible, organize petitions, specifying clear demands to improve health and safety, including reducing exposure to dangerous chemicals, substitution of safer chemicals whenever possible, and improving ventilation. In addition, work to have reproductive-safety concerns included in union negotiations or other employee contracts.

7. Learn what information your employer is legally required to furnish you in regard to the reproductive hazards of your workplace. Your local department of labor, your union, NIOSH (the National Institute for Occupational Health and Safety) plus your local state and city coalitions on occupational health and safety can provide the specific regulations your employer must adhere to in regard to your welfare.

YOU ARE NOT ALONE!

If you believe your working environment may be harmful to your fertility—or to any aspect of your health—or if you would like further information on the reproductive hazards of the workplace, the following organizations can help you:

COMPUTER DATA BASES:

Medline	National Library of Medicine, Bethesda, Md. References from over three thousand biomedical journals can help you zero in on the specific health hazards of your job
Toxline	National Library of Medicine, Bethesda, Md. Four hundred thousand references on human and animal toxicology
Toxnet	National Library of Medicine, Bethesda, Md. A toxicology data bank
Reprotox	Reproductive Toxicology Center, Washington, D.C. Referenced summaries of more than seven hundred reproductive toxins

HOTLINE ORGANIZATIONS

For additional written material and/or references to help in your area or occupation, contact the following organizations:

9 to 5
National Association of Working Women
614 Superior Avenue, N.W.
Cleveland, OH 44113
(216) 566–9308

National Network to Prevent Birth Defects
Box 15309, S.E. Station
Washington, DC 20003
(202) 543–5450

Safe Company, Inc.
368 Hillside Avenue
Needham, MA 02194
1–800–222–3003
In Massachusetts: (617) 444–7778
Provides free information on Safe Monitor.

Occupational Safety and Health Administration (OSHA)
U.S. Department of Labor
200 Constitution Avenue NW
Washington, DC 20210

There are also regional and local state offices. OSHA will perform workplace inspections at request of an employee, a union, or a physician.

National Institute for Occupational Safety and Health (NIOSH)
101 Marietta Tower
Atlanta, GA 30323

There are also local state offices. NIOSH investigates health and safety hazards in the workplace, upon request.

Office of Technology Assessment
U.S. Congress, Washington, DC 20510

Provides literature on reproductive hazards of the workplace.

• 6 •

THE FERTILITY PROTECTION UPDATE

A Couple's Guide to a Healthy Lifestyle

*E*very day, it seems, we discover not only new fertility threats, but new dangers in factors that have been present in our lives for a long time. To name just a few:

- ◆ Alcohol
- ◆ Diet pills
- ◆ Tranquilizers
- ◆ Caffeine
- ◆ Pesticides
- ◆ Air travel
- ◆ Acne medications

- ◆ Tobacco
- ◆ Heating pads
- ◆ Electric blankets
- ◆ Cleaning fluids
- ◆ Toaster ovens
- ◆ Color televisions
- ◆ Recreational drugs

In just the past several years, all these have been found to place male and female reproductive health at risk, and the list seems to grow almost every day.

The good news is that the same research that has helped us identify potential dangers to your fertility has also provided ways you and your partner can protect your reproductive health, often just by making a few simple modifications in the course of your daily living. To help get you and your partner thinking in the right direction, I have prepared a short Lifestyle Fertility Quiz, based on information from worldwide studies on reproductive health, as well as important insights provided by my patients and my own observations.

THE LIFESTYLE FERTILITY QUIZ

Each of the following twenty-four statements was designed to help you and your partner learn something about a particular aspect of your lives. The connection between the questions and the subject of fertility is sometimes obvious; at other times the significance of your responses will be more subtle. For this reason, I ask that you both answer each question spontaneously and then go on to the next, without stopping to wonder what your answers mean. The Fertility Scorecard at the end of the test will help you understand the meanings of your responses, as well as providing some important information on the current status of your reproductive health.

To take the test, simply read each statement and then record how true it is for you, indicating *A* for always, *S* for sometimes, and *N* for never. Keep a numbered list of your answers. The same format is followed through the quiz.

	Always	Sometimes	Never
1. I drink more than four cups of coffee a day.			
2. I drink more than two cans of cola a day.			
3. I take pain relievers regularly— more than thirty tablets monthly.			
4. I smoke at least one pack of cigarettes a day.			
5. I need at least two alcohol drinks every day to relax.			
6. I drink more than ten beers or ten glasses of wine a month.			
7. I use marijuana more than once a week.			
8. I use cocaine and/or crack more than once a month.			
9. I have trouble falling asleep at night.			

	Always	Sometimes	Never
10. I have trouble remaining asleep and wake frequently during the night.			
11. I take a lot of over-the-counter medications.			
12. I spend more than twenty hours per week at a computer.			
13. I hate my boss.			
14. I watch more than twenty hours of color TV a week.			
15. My job requires that I be exposed to radiation and/or chemicals on a regular basis.			
16. I fly more than eight hours a month.			
17. I spend most of my time out of doors in a major city.			
18. a. *For women only:* My menstrual cycle is irregular.			
b. *For men only:* My sex drive seems less intense than before.			
19. I exercise more than five hours a week.			
20. a. *For women only:* I use an IUD for birth control.			
b. *For men only:* I take medication for high blood pressure.			
21. I have at least three different sex partners in the course of a month, or I have had multiple partners in the past.			
22. a. *For women only:* I have had problems getting pregnant in the past, or I have never been pregnant.			

	Always	Sometimes	Never
b. *For men only:* Past partners have had difficulty in getting pregnant; I have never impregnated a partner.			
23. I live in a warm climate.			
24. There are bitter odors in the air I breathe at home or at work.			

To score your Fertility Lifestyle Quiz, simply total your *A*'s, your *S*'s, and your *N*'s, assigning them points as shown below:

A responses 10 points each
S responses   5 points each
N responses   2 points each

Add your total score, and then use the Fertility Scorecard to determine the current status of your reproductive health.

FERTILITY SCORECARD

50–100 points: Your fertility is likely in good shape, or at least your lifestyle habits are not making significant contributions to future problems. It is also likely you are a well-balanced person who does everything in moderation. If you maintain your current lifestyle, it's likely you will preserve your fertility and your sex life for many years to come.

101–150 points: You're not quite as careful as you would like to think! While your reproductive health is probably not in any imminent danger, if you keep on doing what you're doing, or add a few more excesses, you may find your fertility in trouble within the next few years. Turn to the Fertility Protection Update in the next section to find out where you need to make some changes.

151–200 points: You are in the danger zone! If you're not having problems conceiving, it's probably because you haven't tried! This high score should tell you that changes need to be made if you want to preserve both your fertility and your sex life for the coming years. Do read the next section, and make important changes right away.

201–250 points: You are in serious danger. Not only is your fertility being jeopardized, but your general health is in trouble as well. If you are able to conceive, your chance of miscarriage and/or birth defects is probably higher than average. If you are also above age thirty and have been living this way for some time, you are at especially high risk for infertility or a problem pregnancy. Read the next section and begin immediately to make some important changes in the way you live, work, and play.

THE FERTILITY PROTECTION UPDATE

Because your reproductive health is a cumulative biological condition, how much or how little your lifestyle influences your fertility has much to do with how long negative aspects have been present in your life and to what degree they are present now. It's important to remember, however, that there are exceptions to all rules. Some men and women continue to be fertile and produce healthy children despite being in poor health themselves or indulging in practices and habits that are detrimental to most people. At the same time, some couples who scrupulously avoid anything that could harm their fertility find they cannot conceive. Science, it seems, can show us the smartest course of action, but nothing can give us guarantees.

With this in mind, I have prepared this Fertility Protection Update, a guide to what the latest research shows will and won't affect your reproductive health. By checking the guide here for factors present in your lives, you and your partner can determine where important changes can be made.

The factors are listed in alphabetical order, and placement does not indicate ranking either of their ability to harm you or of the degree of damage they will cause. How much or how little each factor affects you can vary greatly, depending on the number of negative factors present in your life.

FACTOR: AIR TRAVEL

Effects on Fertility:

FEMALE: A number of important studies have shown that female flight attendants have high rates of irregular ovulation, difficulty in conceiving, and miscarriage. The latest research reports that these may be linked to exposure to high levels of atmospheric radiation.

MALE: Since sperm is exceptionally vulnerable to the effects of all radiation, it is believed that excessive air travel could cause a number of sperm abnormalities, including:

- Decrease in sperm count
- Increase in the number of abnormal sperm
- Sperm too immature for fertilization

For Maximum Fertility Protection:

Avoid all unnecessary air travel for three to five months prior to attempting conception, and avoid as much as possible all air travel during the duration of your pregnancy. Since, in order to save fuel, planes now fly at a higher altitude (where radiation is higher), your fertility may be in more danger than ever before. When this risk is combined with the dangerous effects of x-ray equipment used by airport security, continual air travel can represent a major reproductive threat. This is especially important if you are already at high risk for infertility and/or if you currently have irregular menstrual cycles or a history of miscarriage.

FACTOR: ALCOHOL

Effects on Fertility:

FEMALE: Although your reproductive system is generally less sensitive to the effects of alcohol than your partner's, a number of studies report that even drinking in moderation can cause menstrual disorders leading to infertility. An important new study from the University of Washington reveals that taking even one drink a day several weeks prior to getting pregnant may increase your risk of delivering an exceptionally small, low-birthweight baby, which can have far-reaching health effects throughout your child's life. This can also be crucial if you deliver even a few weeks premature.

MALE: The male reproductive system is extremely vulnerable to the effects of even moderate alcohol intake, with problems rising in direct proportion to how much, and for how long, a man drinks. Chronic alcoholism can result in permanent impotence by affecting the spinal reflex center, the area that controls both erection and ejaculation. When drinking continues long enough, the damage becomes permanent, even after years of sobriety.

Alcohol consumption of just three drinks per day (whether wine, beer, or liquor) can

- ◆ Cause multiple endocrine abnormalities
- ◆ Decrease testosterone levels
- ◆ Increase number of abnormal sperm
- ◆ Lower sperm count

Alone or in combination, any of these can cause infertility. In addition, new animal studies have shown that males that were given alcohol before mating with alcohol-free females produced a greater number of stillborn offspring, as well as offspring that were smaller and more frail.

For Maximum Fertility Protection

In both men and women, even moderate drinking can deplete key nutrients and upset the vitamin–mineral balance. This can, in some individuals who are already malnourished due to dieting or poor eating habits, cause at least a temporary bout with infertility. If you do drink alcohol regularly, follow the fertility vitamin–mineral guide in Chapter Eleven.

To help ensure your fertility, you and your partner should *limit* alcohol intake for at least one month prior to attempting pregnancy. If you are already having problems conceiving, and/or have a history of miscarriage, you and your partner should *avoid all alcohol for at least forty-eight hours prior to conceiving.*

FACTOR: COLOR TELEVISIONS

Effects on Fertility:

MALE AND FEMALE: Like microwave ovens and VDTs, color televisions emit low levels of non-ionizing radiation. Although not considered a prime risk for fertility, when combined with other threats, including exposure to other sources of radiation, the effects can be cumulative and eventually contribute to reproductive problems, including egg damage, ovulation and/or menstrual irregularities, and lowered sperm count.

For Maximum Fertility Protection:

Color television sets manufactured after 1975 emit much lower levels of radiation than those sold prior to that year. However, studies connecting fertility problems to color television sets manufactured after 1975 are still ongoing.

If you watch a lot of TV and you also spend time around other non-ionizing radiation sources, take an extra measure of fertility protection by sitting at least ten feet from your set when watching. This will minimize the effects of radiation.

FACTOR: HOUSEHOLD CLEANERS

Effects on Fertility:

MALE AND FEMALE: While most people are concerned with pollution in the air outdoors, a recent study by the Environmental Protection Agency (EPA) found that the levels of a dozen or more pollutants can be two to five times greater inside the home than outside. The likely culprit: chemicals found in household cleaners:

- ◆ Rug or upholstery shampoo
- ◆ Furniture polish
- ◆ All-purpose cleansers
- ◆ Pesticides (for example, roach spray)
- ◆ Bathroom cleaners
- ◆ Room deodorizers

Since manufacturers of these items are required by law to list only those ingredients that have been proved hazardous (most of which are innocuously identified as "poisons" or "irritants"), it's difficult to say with certainty which of these products can affect your reproductive health. However, many contain substances that have been shown to decrease fertility in men and women alike, especially

- ◆ Organic solvents (such as benzene)
- ◆ Petroleum distillates
- ◆ Formaldehyde

For this reason, you should minimize your use of all chemical products and certainly not use any to excess for at least several months prior to attempting conception. Once you *are* pregnant, observe extreme caution regarding use of these items.

FACTOR: LOW-VOLTAGE APPLIANCES

This category includes heating pads, electric blankets, toaster ovens, clock radios, and so on.

Effects on Fertility:

MALE AND FEMALE: It has long been known that exposure to high-voltage sources of electrical current (like those emitted from high-power lines) can have detrimental effects on your fertility. It was recently learned that continual exposure to even low-voltage appliances can have detrimental effects on fetal development. In addition, studies show that the temperatures of some heating pads may damage your eggs, upset ovulation, and decrease your conception odds, and they may decrease sperm count and quality in your partner.

For Maximum Fertility Protection:

If you are trying to conceive, don't use a heating pad, especially in your genital area. If you normally use this appliance for menstrual cramps try a hot water bottle instead, or one of the new microwavable heat packs. Use these items for as short a time span as possible.

In addition, if you are trying to get pregnant, and especially if you have already conceived, remain at least six feet from any low-voltage appliance in use. If your alarm clock is electric, make certain it is at least at an arm's-length distance from your bedside, and don't sleep under an electric blanket.

FACTOR: MEDICATIONS

Effects on Fertility:

FEMALE: Generally speaking, when properly used, most medications will not interfere with your ability to get pregnant. However, because everyone's body responds to drugs uniquely, it's sometimes difficult to predict the reaction of your reproductive system to medication. For this reason, always advise your gynecologist-obstetrician of any drugs you are taking on a regular basis (whether prescription or over-the-counter), including:

- Allergy pills
- Pain relievers
- Cold remedies
- Tranquilizers
- Cough medicines
- Antidepressants
- Gastrointestinal aids
- Antibiotics

In addition, you must mention if you are on medication for chronic illness, such as diabetes, heart problems, high blood pressure, kidney ailments, or arthritis.

Since many drugs on the market today can cause a variety of birth defects if they are in your system at the time when you conceive, it is vital that you check with your physician about medications you are taking during the time you plan to get pregnant. Ask about eliminating all unnecessary medication for at least one month prior to attempting conception.

MALE: The same general advice applies to your partner. This factor can have an even greater impact on men, since the residues of every drug a man takes pass through his reproductive tract before leaving his body. In addition, the following medications are known to cause fertility problems in men:

◆ Clonadine and other blood pressure medications can cause a decrease in sex drive and temporary impotence.
◆ Chemotherapeutic agents can cause injury to the testes, resulting in sterility.
◆ Methotrexate, used in the treatment of psoriasis and cancer, can cause damage to the testes and stop cell growth.

The following drugs have been reported to lower sperm count and can also cause many other fertility problems, especially for men who might already be experiencing some sperm-related difficulties:

◆ Cimetidene (Tagamet), used in the treatment of duodenal ulcers
◆ Salicylazosulfapyridine (SASP), used in the treatment of irritable bowel symdrome
◆ Phenytoin, used in the treatment of seizures
◆ Sulfasalazine, used in the treatment of ulcerative colitis
◆ Colchicine, used in the treatment of gout

While the subject is seldom discussed, according to a report in the *Journal of Urology* as early as 1974, overuse of penicillin and tetracycline can also depress sperm production.

For Maximum Fertility Protection:

Because many medications work by accumulating in the body, some can remain in your system for as long as a month after the last dose is taken. While they may not directly affect your ability to get pregnant, their presence in your body could affect the quality of your conception. Sperm tainted with drug residue can be generally unhealthy and could impede or even block a healthy fertilization.

For this reason, you and your partner should consult your physician about ways to clear your system of any unnecessary medications for at least one to two months prior to attempting conception.

FACTOR: MICROWAVE OVENS

Effects on Fertility:

MALE AND FEMALE: Prior to 1976 improper manufacturing techniques allowed some microwave ovens to leak questionable amounts of non-ionizing radiation, the effects of which have been associated with incidence of cancer, nervous disorders, and sterility both in men and in women. Today, oven doors are sealed shut, and dangerous leakages are almost nonexistent. However, since the overall effects of non-ionizing radiation are still being investigated, anyone having difficulty conceiving should avoid direct or constant exposure to microwave ovens.

For Maximum Fertility Protection:

Limit use of microwave ovens if you have any of the following:

- ◆ Menstrual irregularities
- ◆ Ovulation difficulties
- ◆ Trouble conceiving
- ◆ A history of miscarriage

If you must use a microwave oven, stand at least six to ten feet away from the unit while it is on.

Since sperm production and quality are extremely sensitive to the effects of all types of radiation, men, even more than women, must obey microwave precautions.

Various types of home testing kits are available to help determine if your microwave is emitting any dangerous radiation. Periodic checks can be one way to ensure that your fertility is not being compromised.

FACTOR: ORAL CONTRACEPTIVES

Effects on Female Fertility:

While there has been much speculation as to whether your fertility is compromised directly following the use of birth control pills, the latest studies report that once discontinued, oral contraceptives provide no negative side effects on your ability to get pregnant. They do, however, cause a slightly higher risk of birth defects, should a pregnancy occur while pill residues are still in your body. Since it can take up to one month or more to fully clear your system of all traces of oral contraceptives, it's a good idea to use another form of birth control for at least two to three months following cessation of the pill, before getting pregnant.

For Maximum Fertility Protection:

The new triphasic birth control pills, which vary the dosage of hormones during the month, have recently been implicated as a possible factor in ovarian cysts. Although studies are still inconclusive, if you have a tendency toward this problem, especially if you have polycystic ovarian disease, you should avoid using this form of birth control to delay pregnancy.

FACTOR: PESTICIDES, FUNGICIDES, INSECTICIDES

Effects on Fertility:

MALE AND FEMALE: Sinice its creation in 1970, the EPA has banned twenty-six pesticides, fungicides, and insecticides. Yet by 1982, 880 million pounds of toxic chemicals were still being routinely sprayed on the most commonly eaten fruits and vegetables, including tomatoes, apples, onions, potatoes, grapes, melons, lettuce, celery, carrots, broccoli, oranges, and peaches. Currently seventy pesticides, insecticides, and fungicides that are actively in use have proved to be carcinogenic in animal studies, and evidence mounts daily for similar effects in humans.

When ingested in the form of residues, these toxic chemicals can:

- Disrupt the functioning of the hormones that regulate the nervous system
- Cause abnormal cell division
- Interfere with the replication and repair of genetic material
- Increase the risk of congenital malformations (birth defects)

Also, when they are present in your body (either through inhalation or from toxic residues left on food), your breast milk can be contaminated, leading to kidney damage, depressed immune system function, and cancer in a baby you breastfeed during this time.

Although studies connecting these toxic chemicals and fertility are just getting underway, preliminary results indicate many can cause

- Menstrual irregularities
- Decreased fertility in men and women
- Impotence
- Decreased sex drive in men and women
- Reduced sperm count
- A high percentage of abnormal sperm

For Maximum Fertility Protection:

Avoid all fruits and vegetables treated with toxic chemicals, and whenever possible purchase foods that are organically grown. Also, look for certification by a California-based company called NutriClean, which tests foods for chemical residues and certifies those that are pure.

Carefully wash all fruits and vegetables before cooking and especially before eating raw. Use a brush, hot water, and a mild soap.

If you live in an area that is routinely doused with pesticides, and especially if you are having trouble getting pregnant and/or have been plagued with repeated miscarriages, you may want to consider relocating before conceiving.

FACTOR: BODYBUILDING STEROID DRUGS

Used for bodybuilding and sports stamina, they are known on the athletic circuit as roids or juice. Common brand names are Anavan and Maxibolin.

Effects on Fertility:

FEMALE: Used even on a temporary basis, bodybuilding steroids can cause

- ♦ Menstrual irregularities
- ♦ Lack of ovulation
- ♦ Cessation of menses
- ♦ Permanent infertility

MALE: In addition to causing heart problems, deep depression, excessive rage, and psychosis, bodybuilding steroids taken on a regular basis can cause

- ♦ Testicle atrophy (testicles shrink in size and can deteriorate)
- ♦ Drastic reduction in sperm count
- ♦ Complete inability to make sperm
- ♦ Sterility

For Maximum Fertility Protection:

Although male fertility problems resulting from steroid use can sometimes be reversed when the drugs are discontinued, these substances can cause dangerous psychological and biochemical changes. They are rapidly addictive and can be deadly, so they should be avoided at all costs. If a man is already using steroids, he should stop at least three months prior to trying to conceive a child, and allow his body to cleanse itself of all steroid residues.

Even more important: In almost every instance, damage to female fertility caused by bodybuilding steroids is irreversible, so *women should never use these substances under any circumstances.*

FACTOR: TOBACCO

Effects on Fertility:

FEMALE: Although it is the nicotine component of smoking that has garnered much of the negative attention in the last decade, cigarette smoke actually contains several hundred potentially dangerous substances, including many carcinogens and mutagens like benzene. In fact, the full range of what a single cigarette contains isn't known because the law does not require that manufacturers disclose this vital information.

At any rate, studies do show a clear reduction in your fertility if you smoke. In addition, your risk of infertility increases in direct proportion to the number of cigarettes you smoke, with the most significant damage reported starting with sixteen cigarettes per day. In addition, the younger you are when you start smoking, the greater your chance of suffering at least some type of smoking-related fertility problems. According to the most recent studies:

- Women who smoke are 3.4 times more likely to take one year or longer to conceive than women who do not smoke.
- The fertility of light smokers (fewer than twenty cigarettes a day) was 75 percent that of nonsmokers.
- The fertility of heavy smokers (more than twenty cigarettes a day) was 57 percent that of nonsmokers.
- The overall rate of pregnancies per cycle was only 22 percent in smokers, compared to 32 percent for nonsmokers.

It is believed that smoking harms your fertility by affecting the inside of your fallopian tubes. This in turn leads to difficulties in egg transport, implantation, delivery to uterus, and transport timing. Any one of these can not only affect your ability to get pregnant, but also increases your risk of tubal inflammation and infection and, consequently, ectopic pregnancy, which is the leading cause of maternal death. In a study of 1,108 women by the World Health Organization it was learned that smokers had higher rates of ectopic pregnancy overall.

Fortunately, stopping smoking can diminish fertility risks associated with cigarettes.

MALE: The negative effect of cigarette smoking on a man's fertility is equal to that of women. With as few as sixteen cigarettes a day a man can experience

- Decrease in sperm count
- Increase in the number of abnormal sperm

- Increased risk of miscarriage in partner
- Increased risk of birth defects
- Decrease in the number of motile sperm
- Decrease in the ability to fertilize an egg

In animal studies it was learned that exposure to nicotine, cigarette smoke, and/or polycyclic aromatic hydrocarbons can

- Cause testicular atrophy
- Block sperm manufacture
- Alter the quality of sperm

In both animal and human studies it has been shown that risks increase in direct proportion to the number of cigarettes smoked.

For Maximum Fertility Protection:

In a new study emerging from Sweden it was learned that prenatal exposure to cigarette smoke could make your baby more susceptible to contracting various cancers later in life. Cigarette smoke can also lead to abnormal placenta implantation and premature labor. Since very often you may be pregnant for weeks before you are aware of it, if you are trying to conceive, both you and your partner should not only avoid smoking but smoke-filled environments as well. The effects you can suffer from second-hand smoke have recently been documented as presenting nearly as great a health risk as that from smoking itself.

FACTOR: X-RAYS

Effects on Fertility:

MALE AND FEMALE: Heavy exposure to the ionizing radiation of x-rays can have major mutagenic effects on the reproductive organs of men and women alike, causing both biological and genetic damage. A man's testes and woman's ovaries can both undergo severe damage with even minimal exposure, including:

- A change in the genetic material present in sperm and egg, increasing the risk of miscarriage and birth defects
- Genetic effects that can inhibit the ability of the sperm and the egg to be fertilized

These can have a profound effect on fertility, in many cases rendering you or your partner sterile. The testes, in fact, are so sensitive to the effects of radiation that even small amounts can bring about serious damage.

In addition, adults who were exposed to a great deal of x-ray radiation as children can give birth to babies with a higher incidence of chromosomal abnormalities and Down's syndrome, a form of mental retardation.

For Maximum Fertility Protection:

Because the effects of radiation are cumulative, the more exposure you have, the greater the risk of reproductive damage, especially if your genitals are directly in the line of the x-ray beams. For this reason, a lead apron should always be used to protect your reproductive organs whenever any type of x-ray is taken.

In addition, any woman of childbearing age who must undergo a diagnostic pelvic or abdominal x-ray should, if possible, have it during the first ten days following the start of a menstrual cycle. This will help prevent any newly fertilized egg from receiving x-ray exposure.

Finally, whenever possible, choose an ultrasound sonogram or an MRI scan in place of an x-ray.

DRUG ABUSE AND YOUR FERTILITY

Currently it is estimated that 5 to 10 percent of all women of childbearing age use illicit drugs or abuse prescription medications like tranquilizers or barbiturates. The statistics for men are equally alarming. Although the reproductive risks of any drug largely depend on the substance itself and the individual way your system metabolizes it, several other factors combine to determine the risk to your fertility:

- ◆ Extent of drug use
- ◆ Amount of the drug used
- ◆ Frequency of use
- ◆ Amount of active ingredients and contaminants
- ◆ Age of the user
- ◆ Length of time the drug is used

Regardless of the substance involved, potential damage does increase with frequency. A single dose of any drug will not be likely to cause your reproductive system any damage, whereas regular or habitual use can be extremely harmful. The younger you are, the more potential reproductive damage you can experience.

HOW DRUGS CAN HARM YOUR FERTILITY

The list of substances that are being abused grows almost daily. Currently it includes illegal street drugs such as:

- ◆ Cocaine   ◆ Crack   ◆ Heroin
- ◆ LSD   ◆ Ecstasy   ◆ PCP and THC

Unfortunately this list has also come to include many "legal" drugs that when taken under medical supervision would be extremely helpful. These include:

- ◆ Tranquilizers (like Valium, Librium, Xanax)
- ◆ Barbiturates (like Seconal, Tuanol, Quaalude)
- ◆ Antidepressants (like Elavil, Tofranil, Asendin)
- ◆ Amphetamines (like dexedrine, biphetamine)
- ◆ Opiates (like morphine, Demerol, Dilaudid)

Because the effects of most of these substances are achieved by creating changes in brain chemistry, it is widely believed that, when abused, they can affect fertility by altering the brain chemistry responsible for the output of reproductive hormones, causing changes in libido, sexual dysfunction, inhibition of cell division, and infertility.

In addition to the long-term consequences of chronic drug use, many substances can have an immediate effect on fertility, lasting up to twenty-four hours. That means if you use certain drugs the day before you

---

THE MOST COMMON PRESCRIPTION DRUGS TO CAUSE BIRTH DEFECTS

In addition to causing conception problems, some of the most commonly prescribed tranquilizers and sedatives can, when used *during* pregnancy, cause your baby harm:

- ◆ Valium: causes cleft palate
- ◆ Quaalude: causes musculoskeletal defects, cardiac and circulatory problems, cleft lip and palate, dislocated hips
- ◆ Xanax: causes assorted congenital anomalies
- ◆ Librium: causes neonatal depression, "floppy baby" syndrome
- ◆ Elavil, Tofranil, Asendin and other tricyclic antidepressants: cause face, head, limb, and central nervous system defects, newborn withdrawal symptoms.

In addition, many street drugs can have similar effects when used during pregnancy.

conceive, and especially an hour or two before, you might be compromising your fertility.

When drugs, whether in your body or in your partner's, don't stop you from getting pregnant, they will almost assuredly have an effect on your conception, possibly causing improper implantation and increasing the risks of miscarriage and congenital malformations (birth defects).

THE ENVIRONMENT AND YOUR FERTILITY

One of the most controversial environmental prophecies concerns the Greenhouse Effect, the heating up of our atmosphere due to pollution from industry, automobile exhaust, and the burning of the rain forests. Because they release inordinately high levels of carbon dioxide, which traps and holds heat that would normally be recycled into space, many scientists contend that these factors are causing the earth to grow dangerously warmer.

HOW CLIMATE CAN AFFECT CONCEPTION

In a recent joint study conducted by the Chemical Industry Institute of Toxicology and Glaxo Inc., Research Park, North Carolina, in conjunction with the Fertility Institute of New Orleans and the Fertility Center of Louisiana, it was learned that sperm undergoes an annual reduction every summer, due primarily to a rise in temperature. In addition, summer weather induces

- ◆ Depression in semen quality
- ◆ Low sperm concentration
- ◆ Fewer sperm per ejaculate
- ◆ Lower percentage of motile sperm
- ◆ Higher percentage of abnormal sperm

Other studies on female fertility have reported that women who live in warmer climates generally have an early menopause, with a premature end to their childbearing years. They also have a higher rate of pregnancy complications and problems with delivery timing when the first trimester of pregnancy takes place in summer months (a spring conception).

If the Greenhouse Effect should accelerate, infertility will continue to rise, and there will be fewer months conducive to pregnancy and fewer areas of the world at optimum conditions for conception.

THE TIME TO PROTECT YOUR FERTILITY IS
RIGHT NOW!

One important misconception about infertility is that it only happens to "older" people. Actually, lifestyle and other problems linked to infertility can begin to affect you almost any time after puberty. In fact, the latest studies show the following:

- Teens, and especially preteens, who smoke experience more fertility problems in later years than do nonsmokers
- Drug abuse in teenagers can inhibit the release of the hormone GnRH. When this occurs, the entire reproductive system may never fully develop.
- Teenagers have the greatest risk of contracting a fertility-robbing STD, with incidence of PID highest for teenage girls.
- The younger a girl is when she begins heavy physical workouts, the greater her chance of permanent infertility.
- Teenage girls and young women who diet and/or are continually underweight risk permanent destruction of their menstrual cycle.

Indeed, the effects of many of the reproductive villains you are reading about in this book, such as alcohol, drugs, and nutritional deficiencies, are much more severe, with more devastating permanent results, when experienced by young men and women.

So regardless of your age, don't let your fertility go unprotected.

· 7 ·

THE NEW OB-GYN EXAM

How Your Doctor Can Protect Your Fertility—Right Now!

As your grandmother—or perhaps even your mother—can tell you, yesterday's gynecological exam was not an event most women exactly welcomed. Seldom was there regard for either a woman's dignity or her threshold of pain.

While today's exam still requires that you assume a few positions I'm not sure would qualify as dignified, thanks to new knowledge about how your body works, plus a variety of exciting high-tech diagnostic and treatment techniques, the new gyn exam has made a quantum leap into the future, offering you fertility protection and care that was never before possible.

WHAT'S NEW—AND WHAT IT CAN DO FOR YOU RIGHT NOW!

Of the myriad advances made in gynecology in the past five years alone, perhaps the most beneficial to your reproductive health are the new ways of tracking down even the deadliest fertility threats in their earliest and most easily treated stages—often right in your doctor's office!

What follows is just a partial list of the most important new diagnostics available to help you preserve and protect your fertility.

118

FOR GONORRHEA AND CHLAMYDIA

- First Response, the company that offers home pregnancy tests, is marketing a professional diagnostic kit for gonorrhea that allows your doctor to perform the test right in the office and obtain results in just forty-five minutes, rather than after two to three days.
- Eastman Kodak has devised an in-office testing procedure for diagnosing, among other things, chlamydia, the sometimes symptomless STD that until recently was so frustratingly silent that even laboratories could not track it down.

THE GOOD NEWS ABOUT VENEREAL WARTS

- ViraPap is a new diagnostic test that features a revolutionary method of identifying a number of different strains of the potentially deadly human papilloma virus (HPV). One of these strains is responsible for the fastest-growing threat to your reproductive health: venereal warts (see Chapter Four). Previously diagnosis was usually possible only in the more advanced stages of the disease; however, Vira-Pap not only offers early detection, but the chance to predict who is at high risk for this disease long *before* it even develops.

NEW HOPE FOR CERVICAL CANCER

- The new Pap smear has been computer upgraded in both efficiency and interpretation, making it a more effective test for cancerous and precancerous conditions in your uterus.
- The Cytobrush cell collector, a brushlike device, is quickly replacing the cervical swab in cell collections for Pap smears and other gynecological tests. New studies show that thanks to more effective cell sampling, *early cancer detection almost doubles* when the brush is used.

THE BLOOD TEST FOR OVARIAN CANCER

- CA 125 was originally established to help rule out the possibility of *recurring* ovarian cancers. However, new ways of interpreting test results enables the CA 125 to *identify* the presence of cancer cells in many types of first-time ovarian cysts. This can often save the cost and time of needless surgery. If cancer is detected, this test, given early enough, could save your life.

THE BLOOD TEST FOR ENDOMETRIOSIS

◆ A new blood test under development at the University of Oklahoma Health Sciences Center in Oklahoma City may help to detect endometriosis even when no symptoms are present. The test measures the level of antibodies in your bloodstream—the same antibodies that are believed to cause endometriosis by attacking the lining of your uterus. Helping to do away with the exploratory surgery currently needed to diagnose endometriosis, this new test has had a success rate so far of 85 percent. It could help to significantly reduce the risk of reproductive damage that often accompanies the later stages of endometriosis.

THE FERTILITY BLOOD TESTS

◆ FSH–LH–Prolactin: Five years ago we had not even identified these reproductive hormones. Today, using blood tests to monitor excesses and deficiencies, we can diagnose related conditions like PMS and menopause, as well as track down some potential causes of infertility.

THE BLOOD TEST FOR MISCARRIAGE

◆ New studies conducted by a team of British researchers have isolated a common factor in the blood of a high percentage of women who miscarry (see Chapter Fourteen). A test based on these findings is currently being developed (and is expected to be widely available soon) to help identify *prior* to conception those women who are prone to miscarriage. Also underway are treatment options and the development of precautionary measures to reduce the risk for those women who do test positive for pregnancy loss (see Chapter Fourteen).

THE NEW TEST FOR UTIs

◆ Currently under development is a brand-new blood test to identify women prone to urinary tract infections (UTIs). One important goal is to discover what makes women susceptible to certain STDs. To this end researchers at Memorial Sloan-Kettering Cancer Center in New York City report that women with a history of UTIs are likely to have one of two closely related blood types: Lewis $a + b -$ or Lewis $a - b -$.

HIGH-TECH MEDICINE—HOW IT CAN HELP YOU STAY HEALTHIER LONGER

Perhaps the most exciting advances in the new gyn exam are related to the high-tech, computerized equipment that has catapulted fertility protection into territories previously visited only in science fiction.

Discoveries in computer science and in medical science have come together to provide a variety of fast, accurate, and easy ways to diagnose everything from endometriosis to fibroid tumors to ovarian cysts before serious damage occurs.

Of these, the three developments that seem to play the biggest role in gyn care are

- ◆ Ultrasonography
- ◆ The ultrasound vaginal probe
- ◆ Magnetic resonance imaging (MRI) scanner

SOUND PROTECTION: THE WAVE OF THE FUTURE

The ultrasonographic (or ultrasound) examination is fast and easy. A hand-held sound wave transducer (about the size of a small microphone) is slowly guided over the appropriate part of your body (for example, your stomach). Sound waves penetrate your skin and bounce off your organs, which electronically echo their size and shape; a computer produces the image on a screen. Although it is completely painless, a sonogram must be performed when your bladder is full.

WHAT MAKES
ULTRASOUND
SPECIAL

> Not only can ultrasonogram pictures distinguish between bone and tissue, between blood and other body fluids, but because they use no radiation they are safer than an x-ray.

Now You Can Avoid Surgery!

By helping to detect the presence of tumors, cysts, and pelvic masses, and allowing us to analyze their size and structure, ultrasonography is helping many women to avoid exploratory surgery. A look inside your body once required a costly hospital procedure and the trauma of an incision; today, a simple ultrasound photo session can often provide your doctor with enough detailed information to make a correct diagnosis or at least to determine more accurately if a surgical procedure is necessary.

Protection with the Vaginal Probe

Newer and even more effective in protecting your fertility is the vaginal probe, a more precise method of gynecological ultrasonography that utilizes a thin, tubelike transmitter covered with a condom; this is slipped inside your vagina and placed right next to your uterus and ovaries. It provides the added advantage of visualizing even the tiniest tumors and cysts, growths that might otherwise be missed in your manual exam. Easier to endure than a regular ultrasound exam (because it does not require a full bladder), the vaginal probe is now being used for

- ◆ Early detection of ectopic pregnancies
- ◆ Confirmation of intrauterine pregnancy
- ◆ Detecting advanced endometriosis
- ◆ Diagnosing uterine cysts and tumors
- ◆ Aspirating eggs from the ovary for in vitro fertilization

A New Test for Ovarian Cancer

The very newest and most exciting use of ultrasound was recently developed at Kings College School of Medicine and Dentistry in London, England, where researchers have devised a new test for super-early detection of ovarian cancer. Called transvaginal color flow imaging, the test utilizes a vaginal probe to conduct an ultrasound scan of the ovaries, looking for resistance to blood flow, which in turn is depicted by a range of colors on a computer screen.

The researchers have found that the blood vessels of malignant tumors show a marked decrease in blood flow resistance, while benign tumors and cysts have good resistance. This new method of scanning can help to distinguish between malignant and benign growths from the moment they are discovered, which, in turn, helps to bypass the normal wait-and-see period of diagnosis and allows immediate treatment of those growths found to contain cancer cells. Together with a traditional abdominal ultrasound exam, also used for detection of ovarian cancer, the transvaginal color flow imaging will be able to save countless lives.

THE NEW IMAGE MAKERS: THE MRI SCANNER

Radiation-free and thus safer than an x-ray examination, the new magnetic resonance imaging (MRI) scanner uses computerized radio waves bouncing off a magnet to create a high-tech photo of any organ in your body. Currently its primary gynecological use is in examining your pelvic region, especially if you have significant pain for which no cause can be found. It has also been extremely helpful in detecting

- Cancer of the uterus
- Ovarian cancer
- Endometriosis
- Prostate cancer in men

The procedure is completely painless, requiring only that you lie completely still on a bed that is wheeled into a large magnetic tunnel. Here the radio-wave "pictures" are formed and relayed to a computer screen.

MRI—A WARNING

Since MRI was only approved by the FDA in the early 1980s, its long-term side effects are not known. For this reason, pregnant women should not undergo an MRI scan except in critical cases.

THE NEW VIDEO SURGERIES

At the same time that video cameras and VCRs were giving home movies a new meaning, they were also invading the world of medicine, helping to bring several diagnostic and therapeutic surgical procedures into the video age. Today, this technology provides an outstanding new way for your doctor to record and keep track of important medical data about you, including the size, shape, and growth pattern of any internal abnormalities that might exist. New instruments designed for this purpose allow your doctor to connect a tiny video camera to special probes, so as to film everything he/she sees.

When this technology is combined with laser surgery techniques, your doctor can perform your operation while watching a video screen. Guided by the picture, he knows precisely where to aim the powerful laser beams.

Currently video surgeries are used to diagnose and treat

- Endometriosis
- Fibroid tumors
- Ovarian cysts
- Pelvic inflammatory disease
- Venereal warts

WHAT MAKES TODAY'S EXAM REALLY NEW

While each technological advance is a welcome addition to modern gyn treatment, perhaps the most important step forward in fertility care is not scientific at all. It didn't come out of a laboratory or a computer bank, and it has no high-tech background. What makes today's gyn exam really different is the attitude of today's gynecologist toward your health care.

THE NEW GYNECOLOGIST—A DOCTOR FOR THE FUTURE

All over the world gynecologists are expanding the boundaries of their treatment to enable them to act as your *primary care physician,* the source and the guide for *all* your health care needs. No longer limiting their expertise to one area of your body, today's gynecologist recognizes fertility and your overall reproductive health as a *total body concept.* This is especially important for young women: studies show that if you are between the ages of eighteen and thirty-five and consider yourself health conscious (watching your diet, exercising regularly, keeping weight in check), you rarely see any doctor other than a gynecologist. However, since many of the first signs of a fertility problem appear in areas other than your reproductive tract, a doctor who limits your exam to your reproductive organs leaves a serious gap in your fertility protection and care. Many potentially damaging threats to your reproductive health can go completely unnoticed until it's too late.

What are some of the "deceiving" symptoms of impending fertility snafus?

- ◆ Stomach or digestion problems
- ◆ Backache
- ◆ Excessive fatigue
- ◆ Vision problems

Your reproductive health—and maybe even your life—could depend on your gynecologist's serving as your primary care physician during your fertile years. This is what one young patient recently discovered when she found herself in a hospital emergency room one cold and rainy night.

WHEN IT'S TIME TO CALL THE DOCTOR: HOW TO TELL

I was finishing up a weekend of emergency room duty when the ambulance brought her in. Obviously in severe pain, she was pale and sweaty and clutching the right side of her abdomen. "The pain is *so* awful," she whispered.

I quickly examined her and ordered a few tests, and within a short time my diagnosis was confirmed. She was suffering from an ectopic pregnancy. In this case the embryo had attached itself inside her fallopian tube. The pain and the problems began when the egg started to grow, straining against the sides of the tube until they were nearly ready to burst.

We rushed her into surgery in time to remove the misguided egg before a rupture could occur.

SHE HAD NO IDEA SHE WAS PREGNANT

By the next morning she was awake and alert and very grateful that we had caught the problem in time. She told me that the pains had been occurring off and on for several weeks and that she had had no idea she was pregnant. When she called her family doctor, he suggested it might be a stomach virus or nervous tension. He told her to eat lightly and try some over-the-counter antacids, advice she had taken right up to the night before.

While thankful I had been there when she needed help, I was angry that her condition had been allowed to go so far. I wondered aloud why this obviously bright young woman had not looked for gynecological care sooner. Her response? "I never thought of calling my gynecologist about a stomach ache," she said quite innocently. "I didn't know I was pregnant, so I didn't think he was the doctor to call."

Her attitude did not surprise me. Many women, young and old, believe that the only time to seek the care of a gynecologist is when you're pregnant or when reproductive health is clearly involved. While this may have been true at one time, it is true no longer.

Today's gynecologist can be a doctor for all seasons, if you are willing to view him or her in this new light.

THE NEW GYN–T.H.E. EXAM: SEVEN STEPS TO BETTER HEALTH CARE

Along with the new attitudes and practices of today's gynecologists, a new kind of gyn exam has been developed, one that's more practical and applicable to your life and your life-style. Not only does it pay a lot more attention to fertility protection, but it offers you a greater degree of overall preventative care. I call today's exam the GYN–T.H.E., short for Gynecological Total Health Evaluation. It involves seven important diagnostic steps, vital to the protection of your reproductive health. Make sure your gynecologist includes these steps in your exam.

STEP 1: THE FIRST EVALUATION

Today's new exam starts with a comprehensive health history—especially vital if you are visiting a new doctor. To help your physician learn as much about you as possible, make a list of the key things you can remember about your mental and physical health, including any major ailments you experienced as a child, such as specific injuries, broken bones, and contagious diseases like mumps, measles, and chicken pox. All can play a role in your future health, especially if you want to get pregnant.

In addition, if you have a complicated health history, especially if it includes one or more hospitalizations and/or surgeries, write a short synopsis of your problems, including the dates you were hospitalized and the treatments you received. Information on how, and for what reasons, you were treated in the past can give your doctor some important clues about your health today.

Your health history should also include the following:

* Any incidence of STDs—or symptoms you might have had, even if you weren't treated
* Any experience with PID, whether or not you were treated
* Any history of emotional problems or drug or substance abuse
* Information on whether you currently use any recreational drugs or are taking any medications
* Information on whether you've ever had a weight problem
* Your pregnancy history, including, if applicable, your inability to conceive, past miscarriages, or past premature labor. Also include family history of birth defects or inherited diseases, either in your background or in your mate's.
* Any serious or chronic health threats that exist now or existed in the past, such as diabetes, colitis, arthritis, high blood pressure, high cholesterol, heart problems

If your doctor does not make you feel comfortable when you give your health history or you don't feel he or she has the compassion or warmth to foster your trust, speak up about how you feel. If your feelings don't change, seek another physician.

STEP 2: THE COMPREHENSIVE BODY EVALUATION—WHAT IT MUST INCLUDE

Your physical exam should begin with a head-to-toe evaluation. Part of the time, a hands-on physical check must be performed in order to detect important physical symptoms. At other times, a simple "eye-on" view of the patient is enough to tell an experienced physician that things are okay.

THE T.H.E. BODY EVALUATION

- ♦ *Neck.* The physician checks for thyroid malfunctions and swollen glands, both linked to conditions responsible for infertility.
- ♦ *Skin and hair.* Tone and condition can be indications of anything from thyroid problems to hormonal disturbances, even serious infections.
- ♦ *Weight.* Because of the links between weight and fertility, keeping accurate records is one way a gynecologist remains actively aware of your fertility status.
- ♦ *Blood pressure.* Although blood pressure itself has no direct link to fertility, levels that stray too far from the norm, either high or low, can be one of the first signs of other conditions that can ultimately affect your chances to conceive.
- ♦ *Abdomen.* Not to be confused with an internal, or pelvic check, an abdominal examination takes place outside the body; the physician checks for any suspicious abnormalities, including lumps, tumors, or protrusions.

Don't Overlook Any Symptoms!

Your total body evaluation should also include a full investigation of any symptoms or complaint you specifically have, no matter how *unrelated* to gynecology it may seem to be. Often symptoms can be deceiving, with the real problem obvious only to the trained eye.

- ♦ Do you suffer from stomach cramps, gas, and constipation? It could be an ulcer or the first signs of endometriosis or ovarian cysts.
- ♦ Is your throat sore, and are you running a low-grade fever? It could be tonsillitis—or signs of an STD.
- ♦ Pains in your lower back, upper thighs or shins? Maybe a result of too many sit-ups—or the beginnings of one of several serious pelvic problems capable of destroying your reproductive health.

The point to remember is that while your gynecologist may not treat every ailment that strikes you, being your primary care physician allows him or her to evaluate any and every symptom you have and determine if, indeed, you need additional care.

STEP 3: THE NEW BREAST CHECK: WHY SELF-EXAMS ARE NO LONGER ENOUGH

Every year 130,000 new breast malignancies are diagnosed in this country. New studies have linked the use of some types of birth control pills with this figure, and that may mean future fatalities will rise even higher. Right now, one out of every ten women will be stricken with breast cancer sometime in her life; one-third of those will die.

While there is no doubt that self-examination is one of the best preventative steps you can take against this catastrophic disease, I firmly believe that the burden of diagnosis must not be yours alone. Your doctor *must* participate in this vital diagnostic procedure, and it must be a part of every new GYN–T.H.E. exam.

If your doctor does not include a breast exam as part of your checkup, find a new doctor. It's that simple and that vital.

BREAST CANCER AND MOTHERHOOD

Recent research has uncovered new, important links between breast cancer and parenting:

◆ Late motherhood increases risks for breast cancer.
◆ Breast feeding reduces them.

Breast Cancer and Your Fertility

Formerly it was believed that any woman even suspected of having breast cancer should not conceive. Because the high estrogen levels of pregnancy are capable of stimulating dormant breast cancer tissue, as well as increasing the spread of existing breast cancer, conception was considered a life threat for these women. While it still may not be advisable in many cases, according to Dr. Philip Kivitz of the Breast Evaluation Center in San Francisco, new studies show us that in certain instances pregnancy *is* okay, providing the cancerous tissue no longer exists. This is another important reason that a breast exam must be part of your gyn care.

STEP 4: THE PELVIC EXAM

Since the pelvic examination still plays a vital role in the fate and future of your reproductive health, it is also a mainstay in the new T.H.E. exam.

In order to ensure that your fertility is protected, the exam should include a check of the following:

- The vulva, the outside portion of your vagina, where the first tell-tale lesions and sores caused by some STDs begin to appear
- The inside of your vagina for additional sores or lesions and for abnormal discharges and/or odors
- The uterus, checking for growths, tumors, cysts, and endometriosis, as well as abnormalities in size and shape. During this portion of the exam your ovaries and tubes should be manually examined as well to ensure that no damage has occurred there.

If any abnormalities are found, your doctor should evaluate them either by means of an ultrasonogram or an MRI scan, or even by means of a laparoscopy.

STEP 5: DIAGNOSTIC TESTS—WHAT YOU NEED, AND WHEN

Regardless of whether any abnormalities are found in your pelvic exam, but most especially if they are, the next step in the T.H.E. exam is a series of vaginal cultures designed to eliminate the most obvious threats to your reproductive health: STDs and cancer. These tests should include:

- *The Pap smear,* still the best preventative step against cervical cancer. Although many doctors advise this test every two years, to maintain your best line of defense, you should be tested every six months, especially if there is a family history of cancer. If any abnormalities are found in this test, it should be repeated immediately. If results are still questionable, a colposcopy (explained later in this book) should be performed.
- *The ViraPap,* for venereal warts. If you are sexually active, this test needs to be taken every six months. If results show you are at high risk for venereal warts, the test should be repeated every four months.
- *The chlamydia culture:* If you have multiple sex partners, pelvic pain or pressure, or an unusual vaginal discharge, or if you are planning to conceive in the near future, this test should also be performed every six months.

STEP 6: THE GYN–T.H.E. BLOOD EVALUATION

In addition to the vaginal tests you receive during your exam, a comprehensive T.H.E. should also include some blood tests, at least on some occasions. What do you need, and when?

- *SMA 12,* a comprehensive blood chemistry test, given at least once a year. Included is a cholesterol check, of utmost importance if you are taking birth control pills, which have been linked to high levels of lipids in blood, the fats responsible for high cholesterol.
- *CA 125:* In the event your doctor discovers a certain type of cyst during your pelvic exam, this test can help rule out ovarian cancer.
- *T3, T4:* These thyroid function tests should be given at least on the initial visit and then repeated every two or three years, or more often if symptoms include lethargy, sudden weight loss or gain, feeling abnormally hot or cold or being anxious, nervous, and depressed, or if you have trouble conceiving.
- *Estrogen, progesterone, FSH, LH:* These hormonal tests should be given if you are suffering from PMS, menstrual disorders, or infertility.

In addition, you should be given blood and urine testing for any specific complaints you bring to your doctor's attention, even if your reproductive system does not seem to be involved.

STEP 7: THE FINAL EVALUATION

Perhaps the most important part of your exam is the time your doctor takes to explain his or her findings to you. Every GYN–T.H.E. exam should conclude with a doctor–patient conference, at which time your physician should inform you of the following:

- If your exam revealed any problems *as well as* any signs of impending disease. If your doctor is suspicious about any aspect of your health, you should be made aware of his or her concerns, especially if your reproductive health and your future ability to conceive are involved.
- Why certain tests have been taken and what your doctor has been looking for.
- When you can expect test results.
- If, based on the exam, there are any signs of symptoms you should watch for.
- If medication has been prescribed, ask specifically what is it for, the side effects you can expect, the warning signs of trouble, and whether or not this prescription has any restrictions in terms of diet and/or other drugs you may be taking. If you drink alcohol, be certain to ask your doctor if this will also affect your medication.

If you don't understand the diagnosis, and especially if you don't understand your problem or why you have it, please ask your doctor to explain the situation in a way you can understand.

A FINAL NOTE OF CAUTION ABOUT YOUR EXAM

Because some doctors believe that only they need to know what's wrong with you, that *your* understanding is irrelevant, they purposely avoid these end-of-exam talks, preferring instead to conclude your visit with assurances and a pat on the head.

This won't do. When it is *your* health, *your* fertility, *your* future on the line, *you* deserve to know and understand all you can about whatever your doctor believes to be true for you.

It's also important that you speak up about any aspect of your treatment or care that you feel is lacking, or about any procedure you feel is unduly painful. Why is this important? If you are in pain, you can tense your body to such a degree that subtle but significant internal symptoms can be missed or mistakenly identified.

One final point to remember: Today's gynecologist must show you that he or she is as interested in preventing problems as in treating them. You must not settle for any physician who offers you less than an equal partnership of quality care.

II

◆

THE FASTEST, EASIEST WAYS TO A SAFE NATURAL CONCEPTION!

◆

· 8 ·

MAKING LOVE AND MAKING BABIES

A Couples' Guide to How Sex Affects Conception

All he has to do is walk in the room and your heart begins to pound. Your breathing may become a little heavier, too, as you begin to feel your body tingle and a surge of energy rush through you. Your face may feel a blush of heat, and if you are very aware, you may even notice a throbbing and a wetness in your genital area as your breasts become warm and hard, your nipples stiff and erect.

These are some of the signs of sexual stimulation, a complex emotional and biochemical reaction that can occur when a woman meets a man to whom she is sexually attracted.

LOVE, SEX, AND GETTING PREGNANT

Although research in this area is just beginning, there is considerable evidence to show that sexual arousal and fertility may be intimately entwined. Basing their theory on observations of animal behavior, in which the desire for sex, by both sexes, is triggered only when the female ovulates, some researchers believe that, on an unconscious level, men and women respond somewhat the same.

Although not consciously registered, men, for example, are thought to instinctively sense when a woman is entering the fertile phase of her monthly cycle. They respond to these silent signals with a distinct series of biochemical changes, some of which stimulate their desire for sex. A woman, in turn, can instinctively sense a man's stimulation and becomes stimulated as well, also responding with an increased desire for sex. This encourages intercourse at the most fertile time, when conception odds are highest. The whole process, say some researchers, forms the basis of procreation as we know it.

Some informal research among my own patient population seems to bear out this sex–fertility theory to some degree:

- *Women say* . . . they feel their sexiest around the middle of their menstrual cycle when, not coincidentally, ovulation is occurring and hormones are in high gear. Needless to say, their fertility is also at its peak.
- *Their partners say* . . . they often feel more sexually stimulated when their wives are ovulating, turned on most, they say, by subtle smells.

Other research has indicated that women who have a regular, satisfying sex life, with intercourse at least once a week, have more regular menstrual cycles and fewer fertility problems than those who don't.

GREAT SEX—LESS STRESS—MORE BABIES!

In addition to stimulating hormone production, a satisfying sex life can also be a wonderful way to decrease physical tensions—and by doing so, helps encourage fertility. How? In much the same way that exercise reduces body tensions that can interfere with hormone production, so can sex. Recent research has shown that the tension-releasing power of just one orgasm can be so great for some people that the effects are twenty times more powerful than the average dose of a tranquilizer like Valium or Xanax!

HOW YOUR SEXUAL RELATIONSHIP CAN ENCOURAGE FERTILITY

In addition to the link between sexual desire and conception, there is also mounting evidence that the quality of our sexual relationships—most especially those that are loving, caring, and emotionally supportive—may also have profound positive effects on our ability to get pregnant:

- Women who have not had a menstrual cycle for years can go into spontaneous ovulation when they fall in love.

◆ Even a chance meeting with Mr. Right can, in some women, have a biochemical effect that sets reproductive action in motion!

Whenever I think of this subject, I recall a particular patient, Marlene, who, for years, suffered from seemingly unexplained infertility. She and her husband were physically fine and a check back into their family and personal health backgrounds revealed no apparent problems, yet she could not conceive. Although she never fully revealed it, I had sensed that her marriage and her sex life were not happy or satisfying—and I suspected this might be behind her reproductive problems.

HE TREATED HER BADLY—AND HER FERTILITY SUFFERED

From the few occasions when Marlene did confide her feelings, I learned that her husband, Bob, was a chronic gambler who drank heavily and could be merciless at times in his verbal abuse of her. I also learned that she had been an abused child, and to escape her parents, she married Bob, her first boyfriend, right after high school. As a result, she never had the opportunity to develop much self-esteem.

The marriage lasted for ten years, but Bob eventually met another woman and left Marlene. For a long while she was devastated, but after some time had passed and she had begun to put the pieces of her life back together, Marlene discovered that her husband's departure had been the best thing that could have happened to her—and her fertility!

GOOD SEX MADE THE DIFFERENCE

Not long after starting a new job in the real estate business, Marlene met Roger, a warm, supportive, and very loving man who encouraged her in every possible way. Thanks to his gentle concern and giving heart, Marlene blossomed. Not only did she return to school and acquire an advanced real estate license, but she and Roger became partners in a real estate business that began breaking sales records in their area. Two years later, they were married. The best news of all: just six months after that, Marlene was pregnant!

HOW LOVE AFFECTS FERTILITY

Although no one can be completely sure that Marlene's body chemistry would not have changed on its own, there is growing evidence that when you feel happy, secure, and loved and have a fulfilling sex life, one that makes you feel good about yourself emotionally as well as physically, your fertility can prosper. How does this happen? As explained more fully in Chapter Ten, your hypothalamus gland, the command center for all your reproductive hormones, is an extremely sensitive barometer of your emotional climate. When you are happy and feel good, it works in peak order. When you are severely troubled, its functions can decrease, and in turn the blood chemistry necessary for reproduction can suffer. Very often unexplained infertility is the result.

Will every romantic disagreement harm your fertility? Probably not. However, if your relationship is chronically stressful, you can experience serious hypothalamic changes, some of which may result in infertility.

GREAT SEX—SUPER FERTILITY: HERE'S WHY!

In addition to keeping your hypothalamus in good working order, an emotionally and physically rewarding sexual relationship can yield yet another important benefit: an increase in your level of endorphins, the chemicals your body manufactures to dull your sense of pain and heighten your ability to experience pleasure.

Not only will this enable you to enjoy sex more, but high levels of endorphins have been found to have a beneficial effect on the ability of the hypothalamus gland to communicate important reproductive signals to the pituitary gland. This, in turn, can result in higher reproductive potential, enabling you to get pregnant faster and easier.

WHEN BAD SEX LEADS TO CONCEPTION

Although Marlene's case is typical of hundreds I have seen over the years, it's important to note that not every woman's fertility is affected by the stress of bad sex. Just as being in a great relationship is no guarantee that you will get pregnant, being in a detrimental one is no promise that you won't. In fact, I have counseled many loving and caring couples who, despite their emotionally sound relationship, suffer from unexplained infertility. I have also seen some of the most disastrous relationships yield a pregnancy and take both the man and woman by complete surprise.

PRACTICAL SEX AND YOUR FERTILITY

Later in this book you will learn how certain sexual positions can influence your ability to get pregnant, and you'll read about the ones to use for a faster, easier conception. But, in addition to this, there are some practical aspects of sex that can affect your fertility, in some cases encouraging conception, in others, not. Here are some of the things that can make a difference if you are trying to conceive.

ORAL SEX

Whether performed occasionally or frequently, oral sex *by* either partner *to* either partner should have no long-term adverse effects on your reproductive health. However, because bacteria normally found in saliva can have some degrading effects on semen, they can reduce its ability to fertilize an egg. For this reason you should avoid having oral sex performed by your partner on you at the time you are trying to conceive.

ANAL SEX

An increasingly popular sexual practice between men and women, when done properly, anal sex can be highly erotic and extremely pleasurable for both sexes. However, if it is performed during the same lovemaking session in which you plan to conceive, an important precaution must be taken. A man must wash his penis with soap and water between acts of anal and vaginal intercourse. Otherwise, harmful bacteria that live in your anus can be transferred into your reproductive tract via your partner's penis. Should conception occur at this time, your newly fertilized egg may be affected.

LUBRICANTS AND CREAMS: WHAT TO USE—WHAT TO AVOID

Many women find that using a lubricant during intercourse makes sex more pleasurable; however, what you use can affect your ability to get pregnant. Oil-based lubricants, such as petroleum jelly or massage oils, can upset the natural pH level of your vagina and create an internal environment that can be so hostile to sperm that it is destroyed before it can reach the egg. In addition, some oil-based products can interfere with sperm activity, decreasing sperm's ability to *swim* through your reproductive system and sometimes even blocking passage to your egg.

To encourage fertility, avoid all products containing a large amount of oil, opting instead for those that are *water* based. (An ingredient label should clearly identify the product's contents or you can look for the statement "SAFE TO USE WITH CONDOMS." Since oil can break down latex, these products are all water based.)

HOW HOT TUBS CAN BLOCK PREGNANCY

While hot tubs are popular for an extremely sensual form of intercourse, in terms of your fertility, the pleasure may not be worth the price:

- The high temperatures of hot tub waters may damage your "egg of the month" and interfere with conception.
- When the temperature of a man's testicles is raised only a few degrees, his sperm count can suffer. Just one lovemaking session in a hot tub, or a soak just prior to intercourse, can damage a man's sperm count and hamper fertility for up to several weeks.

The solution? No hot tubs if you're trying to get pregnant.

CAN A VIBRATOR HARM YOUR FERTILITY?

If used properly (and not shared by others), a vibrator is not likely to have any effect on your fertility, and generally is safe to use at the time of conception. However, viruses and bacteria capable of affecting your fertility can live on a vibrator. If used by someone who is infected, that person's infection can be passed on to you. So, a vibrator that is not hygienic could place your reproductive health in jeopardy.

To properly clean a vibrator, wash it carefully with a sanitary cloth, using hot water and soap—but *do not allow water to get inside the mechanism.*

UNDERWATER SEX AND CONCEPTION

Earlier this year, a patient came to see me when, even after a romantic vacation in the sunny Caribbean, to which she and her husband had gone for the sole purpose of conceiving, she was not able to get pregnant. Although she had no fertility problems to speak of, and her ovulation timing was right on target with her scheduled trip, nature would not comply.

Even with optimum biological and psychological conditions, pregnancy won't *always* occur, of course, but in Katrina's case, I somehow had the feeling there was another force working against her. Questioning her, I soon found out what it was. Katrina and Klaus had taken full advantage of the private pool in their lavish, exotic hotel suite and made love in the water several times a day. In fact, even when their sex occurred elsewhere, it almost always followed a nude dip in their private waters.

Although a sensual experience, making love underwater may not be advantageous for fertility. Not only can water cause a change in the vaginal mucus needed for proper sperm passage, but the chlorine found in most pools can alter your internal pH level and create an environment hostile to sperm.

The next time around, Katrina and Klaus stayed out of the pool—and they conceived almost immediately!

DOUCHING AND YOUR FERTILITY

Generally speaking, the vagina is a self-cleansing organ, with regular, normal secretions that work as a kind of natural hygiene system for internal cleansing. It works equally as well after menstruation and intercourse as it does every day to stay healthy, clean, and free of odors. When odors do appear, they are generally the result of bacteria that reside on the outer portion of the vagina (called the labia) and can usually be eliminated via washing this area with soap and water. Odors can also be caused by infections, which are generally treated with oral medications, or occasionally, a medicated douche.

So, unless recommended by your doctor for specific purposes (we'll tell you more about these in a moment), not only is regular douching *not necessary, but it is also not recommended.* Some studies suggest that it may harm the future of your fertility. How?

Should any bacteria be present in your vagina—as the result of contracting an STD (see Chapter Four), following an abortion, or the insertion or removal of an IUD (see Chapter Two)—douching, especially with a high-pressure force, can quickly drive them into your reproductive tract, allowing faster and easier passage to your cervix and into your fallopian tubes. This, in turn, can increase your risk of PID and its fertility-related consequences (see Chapter Two). The risk of contracting PID increases if you douche before, during, or right after menstruation, when your cervix is in a slightly more open position.

Because of its link to PID, there is some evidence that regular douching may also increase your risk of ectopic pregnancy (see Chapter Two). In at least one study, women who douched once a week had twice the incidence of ectopic pregnancy as those who did not douche at all. Even douching only once or twice a month can be harmful if performed in the week following ovulation.

DOUCHING AND CONCEPTION: A NEW WARNING

In addition to the effects douching can have on the future of your fertility, when performed just before or just after making love, it can also disrupt your immediate ability to get pregnant.

Douching Before Intercourse

Much like the skin on your face and body, the lining of your vagina has a pH reading—an indication of the amount of acid on the surface. Under normal conditions, vaginal pH falls between 4.5 and 5.0, an environment that highly favors sperm. When a normal pH exists, douching just before intercourse can alter your internal environment, causing it to become either too acidic or too alkaline. Either extreme can adversely affect sperm motility and even survival. Unless your doctor diagnosed an abnormal pH balance (you'll learn what to do about that in a moment), douching just prior to attempting conception could adversely affect your ability to get pregnant.

Douching Too Soon After Intercourse

This can wash sperm out of your body that might otherwise have made it to your fallopian tubes. By cutting down on the number of sperm available for fertilization, you can decrease your chance of conception. This can be especially crucial if your partner has even a marginally low sperm count, and/or if your reproductive system contains barriers (such as endometriosis or scar tissue) that can block some of the sperm along the route to your egg.

In addition, I believe that should conception occur, douching too soon after making love, especially with high-pressure apparatus, may have adverse effects on your newly fertilized egg, possibly increasing your risk of miscarriage.

If you find it absolutely essential to douche after intercourse, make certain to wait at least two hours before doing so.

WHEN DOUCHING CAN HELP YOU

Sometimes, because of certain forms of vaginitis (especially a yeast infection) or other biochemical disturbances, the natural pH level of your vagina can be disturbed, making pregnancy difficult and sometimes seemingly impossible. In such cases there are douches that can help.

If you are having trouble conceiving and your doctor diagnoses an abnormal vaginal pH level—either too high, meaning you have too much acid, or too low, indicating not enough acid is present—then one of two natural douches can be used to return the balance to normal.

- ◆ To *reduce vaginal acid:* Use a low-pressure douche of two tablespoons of baking soda in one quart of water just before intercourse.
- ◆ To *increase vaginal acid:* Use a low-pressure douche of two tablespoons of vinegar in one quart of water taken just before intercourse.

In addition, if you are having artificial insemination (see Chapter Nineteen) in place of your douching, your doctor may spray the inside of your vagina with a solution at the proper pH just prior to depositing the sperm. In some cases this may help to increase the rate of pregnancy.

SPECIAL NOTE: Home-douching apparatus, especially the reusable type, can harbor potentially harmful bacteria that are literally sprayed into your body during the douching process. To make certain this does not occur, always properly cleanse all douching apparatus just before use, with lots of soap and hot water.

DOUCHING PRODUCTS: AN IMPORTANT WARNING

Some commercially prepared douches contain ingredients that can harm a developing fetus when used during pregnancy. If you find that you must douche, I suggest you avoid these products, usually identified with a label that reads "Unsafe for Use During Pregnancy," during the time you are trying to conceive as well.

A FINAL WORD: CAN TOO MUCH SEX KEEP YOU FROM CONCEIVING?

While a woman can safely have as much sex as she likes without disturbing her fertility, men are not quite so lucky. In fact, frequent sex can reduce the amount of sperm available for each ejaculation and that can significantly decrease the chance of conception.

The good news: a man's sperm count rebuilds to maximum capacity if he refrains from ejaculating for just forty-eight hours. So avoiding intercourse or masturbation for two to three days prior to attempting conception will ensure that he is at his optimum fertility level.

· 9 ·

BODY FAT, DIETING, AND FERTILITY
How Your Weight Affects Conception

One of the newest ways you can ensure that your body will be biologically ready for a fast and easy conception is to pay careful attention to your weight, especially in the months and weeks preceding the time you plan to get pregnant. In fact, the latest research shows that by reaching the proper weight six months prior to when you want to conceive (we'll tell you how to determine what's right for you, later in this chapter), you can exert an enormous power over your ability to get pregnant, now or in the future.

What's the connection? Although the theory is still brand-new, the latest findings indicate an important link between your levels of body fat and your reproductive hormones—a connection that could play a vital role in conception, as one of my patients recently discovered.

TOO THIN TO GET PREGNANT?

Certain that the success of her modeling career depended on remaining ultraslim, Jan dieted constantly and worked out frantically. Repeatedly ignoring my warnings that her usual 110 pounds was much too low for her tall frame, she sometimes allowed her weight to drop as low as 102 when work became exceptionally demanding.

While her menstrual cycle was always in question (she continually reported scanty bleeding and irregular periods), it wasn't until recently that Jan herself began to see the error of her high-fashion ways.

Although she looked, felt, and indeed was healthy, Jan discovered she was unable to get pregnant. By the time she confided her problem to me, she was in a state of depression. "I can't believe that after a year and a half of trying, nothing is happening," she said.

Since she had been my patient for some years, I was able to reassure her there were no structural problems behind her inability to conceive. She was free of all tumors and cysts, and her organs were in good shape.

However, a series of blood tests revealed what I had warned her about for several years. Jan's low weight had led to a hormone imbalance that nearly shut down her entire reproductive system. Jan was just too thin to conceive a child.

HOW YOUR BODY FAT AFFECTS YOUR FERTILITY

Although research into the connections between weight and fertility is just starting, we believe the key lies not so much in pounds as in your percentage of body fat. Why is this? Each fat cell you retain in your body is a tiny hormone factory. Using a unique biochemical process, it converts certain body chemicals (primarily the adrenal hormone androgen) into estrogen, one of the key hormones involved in egg production and release. In fact, while some estrogen is made in your ovaries, one-third of your body's precious supply—up to 80 percent during peak times of the month—is actually formed in your fat cells.

- The more fat cells you retain, the greater estrogen-making power your body has.

WHAT TURNS FERTILITY ON AND OFF

- Complete hormonal shutdown can occur if your body fat falls just 10 to 15 percent below the norm of 29 percent.
- Even a slight drop in body fat (below 22 percent) can disrupt hormone levels and cause infertility.
- Increasing your body fat by just 10 to 15 percent over 29 percent can also keep you from conceiving, and it can damage the future of your reproductive health.

◆ The fewer fat cells you have, the less estrogen you can make.

But just having estrogen in your body is not enough to ensure conception success. If you are to achieve your maximum fertility potential, your estrogen must be present at a specific level. Whenever that level rises too high or falls too low, as it can when you have too many or too few fat cells, you can have a problem getting pregnant.

WEAK ESTROGEN—STRONG ESTROGEN

According to another theory, all estrogen is not alike. Subdivided by your body into two types, *weak* and *strong*, each must be maintained in certain amounts. Dr. Jack Fishman, professor of endocrinology at Rockefeller University in New York City, holds that when levels of body fat change, the ratio of weak to strong estrogen is disrupted, resulting in a hormone imbalance that can lead to infertility.

THE PROOF IS IN THE PUDDING—AND THE PIE!

Verification of the connection between body fat and fertility was recently provided by two studies performed by Dr. G. William Bates, a prominent professor of obstetrics and gynecology at the Medical University of South Carolina at Charleston. He worked with twenty-nine ultra-slim women, each no more than 91 percent of her ideal weight. All had been infertile for at least four years, and some had undergone fertility treatments with drugs or surgery, to no avail. Each also had a partner whose sperm tested normal.

Dr. Bates' theory was that the percentage of body fat had dropped so low in each of these women that estrogen was in dangerously short supply—*and* affecting all other hormones in the process.

CAN ICE CREAM AND MILK SHAKES MAKE *YOU* MORE FERTILE?

Dr. Bates asked the women to try a high-calorie weight-gain diet, which he believed might raise estrogen levels, put hormones back in balance, and increase conception odds. At this suggestion, three of the participants left the study. The remaining twenty-six, however, gave weight gain a try. Each worked to gain one-half to one pound per week until she reached 95 to 100 percent of her ideal fertility weight.

The result? Once the goal was achieved, ovulation kicked in! Within one to three years following the increase in body fat, twenty-four of the twenty-six became pregnant. The average gain that made the difference? A mere 8.2 pounds! And over 90 percent of the women in the study were able to conceive naturally, requiring neither drugs nor surgery.

THE FOODS THAT
MAKE YOU FERTILE!

Dr. Bates' high-calorie fertility diet for underweight women consisted of generous meals of the following foods:

- Meat
- Pasta
- Whole milk
- Fish
- Cheese

Plus frequent snacking on ice cream, pastry, milk shakes, and beer.

CAN YOU BE TOO FAT TO CONCEIVE?

Just as too few fat cells can upset estrogen levels so, too, can too many, flooding your system with an estrogen overload that upsets timing and function of other hormonal activity. This can result in infertility.

To help verify this, Dr. Bates placed thirteen overweight women—all infertile and averaging 169 pounds—on a diet developed to encourage the loss of about one pound per week. The results?

- An average loss of twenty pounds per woman restored ovulation in eleven cases.
- Ten of the women were able to conceive naturally after losing the weight.

GETTING YOUR BODY READY FOR
PREGNANCY

After I had explained the body fat–fertility connections to Jan, she decided to give weight gain a try. I'm happy to report that just seven-and-a-half pounds and nine weeks later, tests showed that her ovulation patterns and her menstrual cycle were normal, perhaps for the first time in years. Three months after that, she was able to conceive.

To help Jan—and all women—obtain *and keep* the important estrogen-body fat equation in super balance, I believe nature created a woman's anatomy with her reproductive physiology in mind. Your hips were designed to protrude slightly from your body, while your buttocks, breasts, thighs, and stomach were meant to take on a soft, convex shape—no arbitrary decision on nature's part. I believe it is these rounded contours that allow your body to hold sufficient fat necessary for adequate estrogen production. Using your *natural* contours as a guide, never allowing your body to become too fat or too thin, you can not only encourage a fast and easy conception, but help preserve your childbearing options throughout your reproductive years.

FINDING YOUR IDEAL FERTILITY WEIGHT: HOW TO KNOW WHAT'S RIGHT

Until recently, most physicians utilized something called the Metropolitan Height and Weight Standards chart to decide whether a patient was overweight or underweight. With the push toward living on the lean side, however, some health professionals, particularly cardiologists, have begun to think these numbers too high. I, however, along with many other fertility specialists, believe that, at least for the purposes of conceiving, the Metropolitan Standards are correct. Based on these numbers, the chart on page 149 can help you find your ideal fertility weight.

HOW TO CALCULATE BODY FAT LEVELS

Although keeping your weight under control will generally keep your body fat at the right level, too, sometimes pounds can be deceiving. Why? Muscle mass weighs more than fat, so it's possible that you might be at the optimum fertility *weight* but still be short on sufficient body fat. There are a number of sophisticated laboratory tests for determining body fat levels, but there is a simple way you can make your own determinations and monitor levels whenever you want to conceive. The method is called body mass index, or BMI.

MEASURING YOUR BODY FAT: WHAT DO DO

Using metric system measurements, BMI calculations begin with an accurate reading of your weight and your height. Once you have established these figures, you must convert them to the metric system.

1. To convert your weight from pounds to kilograms, divide the number of pounds you weigh by 2.2. For example: weight, 125 lb ÷ 2.2 = 56.8 kg.
2. To convert your height measure from inches to meters, divide the number of inches by 39.4. For example: Height: 60″ ÷ 39.4 = 1.5 meters.
3. You must then *square* your height measurement by multiplying it by itself; in this case, 1.5 × 1.5 = 2.25.

To calculate your percentage of body fat, divide your body weight in kilograms by your squared height in meters. The result will be your BMI. For example: 56.8 Kg (weight) ÷ 2.25 (squared height) = 25.2.

IMPORTANT!
HOW TO FIGURE
YOUR BODY TYPE

To accurately figure which numbers indicate your correct weight, you must determine if you have large bones or small bones. Use this formula:

- Small bones = a wrist measurement of 5½" or less; ankles, 8" or less
- Large bones = wrist measurement of 6" or more; ankles, 9" or more

For small bones, use the lower weight as your guide; for large bones, use the higher weight.

THE FERTILITY HEIGHT AND WEIGHT GUIDE

If Your Height Is:	Your Preconception Weight Should Be:
4'10"	109–121 lb.
4'11"	111–123
5' 0"	113–126
5' 1"	115–129
5' 2"	118–132
5' 3"	121–135
5' 4"	124–138
5' 5"	127–141
5' 6"	130–144
5' 7"	133–147
5' 8"	136–150
5' 9"	139–153
5'10"	142–156
5'11"	145–159
6' 0"	148–162

Note: Height includes 1" heels; weight includes 3 pounds of clothes.

- If your BMI falls between 19 and 25—congratulations! Your body is ready to conceive right now!
- If your BMI is over 27.5, you need to lose body fat before you get pregnant; if it is over 31.5, your loss should be medically supervised.
- If your BMI falls below 19, you need to increase body fat before attempting conception.

ACHIEVING YOUR FERTILITY WEIGHT GOALS

Whether you need to lose or gain body fat, the latest research suggests that *how* you obtain your preconception weight goals can affect your fertility. What should you avoid? Any diet or exercise program that promotes an exceptionally *rapid* gain or loss. Why?

Each significant shift in weight, whether up or down, causes a corresponding shift in hormone production. Because many reproductive functions take their cue from the amount of certain hormones in your bloodstream, levels that change too abruptly can confuse the signals being sent from your brain to your body. The result—your reproductive system falls into biochemical chaos, and you're infertile. Even more important, continual fluctuations in weight keep hormone levels constantly on the move.

Studies show that victims of the yo-yo diet syndrome—hopelessly caught in the lose–gain–lose groove—are at higher risk for reproductive problems when compared with those who lose weight slowly and keep it off. I have observed that many patients who have problems stabilizing their weight also have problems getting pregnant. Even short-term dieting can affect your fertility. Studies at the Institute of Psychiatry in Munich, Germany, recently revealed that if your weight falls within the normal range, trying to lose even a few pounds can cause your menstrual cycle to become so irregular that ovulation is impaired, causing at least temporary infertility.

HOW TO ENHANCE YOUR FERTILITY

The good news is that by following a few simple guidelines, you can *safely* achieve your preconception weight goals and enhance your fertility at the same time! What should you do?

- If you need to lose body fat, eat balanced, nutritious meals of no fewer than 1200 calories a day. Avoid liquid diets, high-fiber quick-loss products, or any diet that utilizes just one food group, such as all-protein or all-vegetable diets.
- If you need to add body fat, add complex carbohydrates (whole-grain pastas, fruits, and vegetables) to your diet, rather than fatty foods, especially those containing tropical oils.

- Avoid all use of diet pills or any commercial weight-loss or weight-gain products. Because every woman's physiology is different, it's difficult to tell if what you are taking could have residual effects on your reproductive system.
- Whether you need to lose or to gain weight, be certain to get adequate amounts of protein every day, at least 46 grams (or about 180 calories). The latest studies show this can help reduce your risk of ovulatory problems.

Finally, remember to give your body adequate time to adjust to your new weight before trying to conceive. In addition to allowing at least one month of dieting time for every six to eight pounds you need to lose or gain, plan on an additional six to eight weeks of maintenance time after you have reached your weight goals *before* attempting conception.

By making sure weight changes are gradual and then giving your reproductive chemistry *time* to readjust, you will not only remain healthy *while* you are dieting, but will also ensure that your body will be in great shape when you reach your fertility weight goals—ready when you are, to conceive and deliver that perfect baby!

• 10 •

FITNESS, STRESS, AND GETTING PREGNANT

Every day I find more evidence that being physically fit *before* you get pregnant can help you have a healthier pregnancy. A patient whose muscles are strong and well toned and whose cardiovascular system is in peak order prior to conception has the best chance of sailing through her pregnancy with few problems; her delivery is likely to be natural and problem-free as well.

However, as beneficial as working out can be to your reproductive health, studies show—and my patients have proved as well—that some strenuous activities work against female fertility. They can cause a variety of negative effects, from menstrual irregularities to outright infertility, for nearly all women of childbearing age. What are these activities? Endurance workouts, including:

- Marathon running
- Excessive jogging
- Frequent high-energy aerobics
- Triathalon training

In fact, studies show that any workout regimen that promotes *extreme* physical and/or emotional stress can be detrimental to your reproductive health. When performed on a regular basis, especially in the months prior to attempting conception, such workouts may seriously reduce your chances of getting pregnant by

- Affecting your ability to produce eggs
- Encouraging irregular ovulation
- Stopping ovulation

If you should conceive, serious implantation problems could result. In some cases, other studies have shown endurance workouts can compromise your fertility to the point of infertility.

HOW YOUR WORKOUTS CAN BLOCK A PREGNANCY

Although no one is exactly sure why endurance sports affect your reproductive health so dramatically, the latest studies point to their influence on your hypothalamus, the gland that secretes gonadotropin-releasing hormone (GnRH), which helps initiate the entire egg production–release process. Some research has shown that workouts that require you to push your body too hard for too long a period of time may inhibit the functioning of your hypothalamus gland, and in the process upset the function of timing of all reproductive hormones necessary for conception.

In addition, endurance training is also thought to alter the way your body metabolizes thyroxin, the hormone produced by your thyroid gland and linked to the reproductive process. Eventually this important gland can malfunction to such an extent your entire body chemistry is adversely affected and your fertility comes to a complete halt.

THE BODY FAT CONNECTION

Even more important are the effects of endurance workouts on body fat, often forcing you to burn massive amounts in a relatively short amount of time. Like strenuous dieting (see Chapter Nine), manic fitness activities can burn so much body fat that your estrogen levels become dangerously low. When this happens, your reproductive system can actually return to a prepubescent stage. I have seen a number of patients who, after losing excess body fat, develop such an irregular menstrual cycle that ovulation eventually stopped. Sometimes it was difficult or even impossible to recharge their reproductive systems and rejuvenate their fertility, even with medication.

A recent study found that marathon runners with continuously low levels of body fat had almost no estrogen in their bodies and consequently had no menstrual cycle. Even after being given estrogen replacement therapy, damage to their reproductive system had progressed to such a degree that the other hormones necessary for conception remained too low for pregnancy to occur.

WORKING OUT: THE SILENT DANGERS

What can complicate things even more is that unlike dieting, where weight change can signal that hormone levels may be dropping too low, the effects of endurance workouts can be dangerously silent. Why? As you lose pounds, you build new muscle mass, which can allow your weight actually to remain the same. Since it is body fat and not just pounds that you need to be fertile (see Chapter Nine) you can be fooled into believing your weight is adequate for optimum fertility, when, in fact, it is not.

Often female athletes with the most severe reproductive problems are near or at their correct body weight. But since that weight is muscle, and not fat, they remain infertile.

Only a small dip in fat stores (just a few percentage points below normal) is enough to trigger menstrual irregularities, so it doesn't take very long for endurance workouts to affect your ability to get pregnant.

SUPER HAZARDS FOR YOUNG ATHLETES

Research shows that the earlier in life you become involved in endurance training, the more likely you will suffer conception-related difficulties and sometimes even permanent reproductive system damage. In fact, each year of endurance athletic training taken prior to puberty delays the onset of the menstrual cycle by an average of 0.4 years. It is not unlikely for some female athletes never to get a menstrual cycle.

In addition, even dancing when done to excess has the potential to harm a young girl. Studies show that some ballerinas who begin rigorous training and/or professional dancing prior to puberty, may never get a menstrual cycle. Many older ballet (and other) dancers lose their menstrual period for months or even years on end while performing on a regular and rigorous schedule.

For this reason I always advise my patients who have young daughters to see that they practice cautious moderation when participating in sports and other demanding physical activities, making sure they cut back whenever any sign of impending reproductive damage becomes apparent—like a delay in the initial onset of the menstrual cycle (past age fourteen or fifteen could be a sign of trouble) or, if they are already menstruating, a cycle interruption of more than three consecutive months. Remember, damage to the reproductive system can occur at almost any age, and it's never too early for a girl to begin caring for her fertility.

HOW EXERCISE CAN PROTECT YOUR FERTILITY: THE GOOD NEWS!

Even with its dangers, there is no doubt that some degree of physical activity is not only safe, but essential to a healthy body. In fact, recent studies have shown that if you are athletically active in your twenties and thirties, you will have a lower lifetime incidence of

- Breast cancer
- Uterine and ovarian cancer
- Cervical and vaginal cancer
- Benign tumors of the reproductive system
- Benign breast disease

The Center for Population Studies at the Harvard School of Public Health recently published findings that show reproductive cancers occurred 2.5 times less often in athletic women than in those who led sedentary lives.

Finally, many types of exercise can help you alleviate tension and stress and thus help keep your hormones in balance and your menstrual cycle regulated. And that's one of the best ways to ensure your reproductive health.

THE WORKOUTS THAT CAN ENCOURAGE YOUR FERTILITY

The key to your workout success depends on the activities you choose, especially if you are planning to conceive in the near future. What kind of exercise should you be doing if you are trying to get pregnant? Doctors and fitness experts alike agree that you can derive great benefits from noncompetitive, mildly aerobic activities that work to condition all parts of your body simultaneously, without placing strain on any particular muscle group. It's also important that you choose activities that can be sustained for long periods of time without exhaustion. These include:

- Swimming
- Dancing
- Bicycling
- Moderate aerobics
- Walking
- Stretching
- Tennis (in moderation)
- Weightlifting

When done in moderation, all these activities can help keep you in great shape *without* disturbing the delicate body chemistry needed for a fast and healthy conception.

HOW YOGA CAN HELP YOU GET PREGNANT

You should also note the positive power that *passive muscle-toning workouts* can have on your ability to get pregnant. Many of my patients have reported great success with yoga, which utilizes a series of body *positions* (rather than *moves*) maintained for increasing lengths of time to condition and tone the body. According to some experts, yoga can help encourage your fertility not only by decreasing stress levels, which in turn can help promote healthier functioning of your hypothalamus, but by having a positive effect directly on your reproductive organs, as the activity increases blood flow and circulation in this area. Studies show that practicing yoga on a regular basis may help promote more regular menstrual cycles, keep reproductive hormones in balance, and alleviate the symptoms of premenstrual syndrome.

If you have never participated in yoga fitness before, you need professional guidance. Books, videotapes, and especially a personal instructor can get you started in the right direction and help you master the postures that encourage fertility.

MAKE ALL YOUR WORKOUTS WORK FOR YOU

Regardless of your choice of activity, you can be sure that your fitness regimen continues to work *for,* not *against,* your reproductive health if you follow a few simple guidelines:

- ◆ Practice moderation. Limit workouts to three times weekly, with at least a day of rest in between.
- ◆ Keep each workout short: no more than forty-five to sixty minutes per session.
- ◆ Avoid becoming *compulsive* about your workouts.
- ◆ Don't let endurance count more than skill.
- ◆ Keep stress out of your workouts by avoiding heavy competition— even with your own records.
- ◆ Don't be afraid to cut back whenever you feel excessive body or brain strain.

Most important, take steps to ensure that your workout is not burning too much body fat. Use the BMI (see Chapter Nine) to monitor levels every seven to ten days, then cut back on activities whenever weight or body fat drops below the accepted norm.

HOW STRESS AFFECTS CONCEPTION

In much the same way that the chronic stress of a bad relationship can affect your fertility, the ways in which your body processes and deals with *all* kinds of stress can have significant effects on your ability to get pregnant now or in the future.

Stress is capable of causing everything from a brief menstrual upset to complete, and sometimes permanent, cycle shutdown. I have personally seen a number of patients whose stress level was so high it represented a serious threat to their fertility.

HOW STRESS CAN BLOCK A PREGNANCY

Because your hypothalamus, the gland responsible for the flow and timing of all your reproductive hormones, is extremely sensitive to both emotional and physical tensions, almost any type of stress has an immediate effect on its functions. That's why your period can be up to two weeks late or even skip a month when you are going through an especially trying time.

Although the effects of short-term stress usually cause only temporary infertility, distress that goes on for long periods of time can have more serious, long-lasting effects. Not only can long-term stress lead to a higher incidence of fertility-robbing diseases, such as endometriosis, vaginitis, and some STDs, but it can throw your reproductive hormones into a biochemical chaos. Often these imbalances cause even more stress, which in turn affects your hypothalamus even further, creating a vicious circle of fertility-related consequences that can ultimately bring your childbearing options to a halt. Sometimes it can be difficult, even impossible, to reverse the damage.

THE GOOD NEWS

The effects of stress can be devastating, but there *is* good news—this is one fertility danger you can control. By keeping stress levels in check and remaining as relaxed as possible in the months and weeks prior to when you want to conceive, you can significantly increase your chances for a fast, healthy conception.

How can you reduce stress in your life? The most obvious way is, of course, to identify the causes and then work to eliminate them from your life. But I do understand this is not always easy or even possible. An irritating boss, disarming in-laws, financial problems, worries and fears about the health of loved ones—these are all *real* problems that we can't escape from. However, if you look into your life, you may see that many of the major stresses are made worse by *smaller* stresses, things you *can* usually control.

If this is the case for you, work to eliminate as many small stresses as you can. When possible, defuse the ones that remain by taking extra time for yourself. The restorative effects of a relaxing herbal bath, a facial or massage, or even a half-hour "me" break, when you can do whatever relaxes *you* (reading a book, window-shopping, gardening, baking) can go a long way in helping you biologically and psychologically cope with stress.

STRESS: THE MOST COMMON CAUSES

While almost anything you personally find stressful can bring about negative changes in your menstrual cycle, the most common major stresses are:

- ◆ Job tensions
- ◆ Relationships with lovers, kids, parents
- ◆ Sexual problems
- ◆ Loneliness
- ◆ Guilt and/or grief
- ◆ Fear of failure
- ◆ Excessive competition

WATCH OUT FOR HIDDEN STRESS

One of the most frustrating aspects of stress is that it can be so deceptive. In our busy lives we can get so used to feeling tense, rushed, fatigued, and even somewhat depressed that we begin to view tension as a normal state of being! Many of my patients don't realize how much tension is present in their lives until a diagnosis of stress-related infertility is made.

For this reason, it's important that you listen to your body for signs of *hidden* stress that could be affecting your reproductive health. The best way to do this is to use your menstrual cycle as a guide. Regardless of how you feel, if you begin to experience irregular cycles (or other possible stress-related menstrual problems, such as cramps, backaches, or sore breasts), arrange for a consultation with your doctor. If hidden stress *is* a problem, he/she can help you uncover the source and map out a plan to reduce tensions. At the same time your doctor can take the *medical* steps necessary to rule out physical problems that may be linked to your stress and help preserve and protect your reproductive health.

HOW STRESSED ARE YOU?

Ask yourself these important questions:

* Am I tired all the time?
* Do I have frequent headaches?
* Do I catch a lot of colds, the flu, sore throats?
* Am I prone to vaginal infections or herpes?
* Is my menstrual cycle irregular?

If you answered *yes* to any of these questions, stress may be a problem. If you said *yes* three times or more, your reproductive health may already be in jeopardy.

AN IMPORTANT WARNING—PLUS, HOW SMILING CAN HELP YOU GET PREGNANT!

Unless your stress levels are exceedingly high and coping is nearly impossible, I do not advise tranquilizers, sedatives, or other medications designed to reduce tension, especially if you are actively trying to conceive. As explained in Chapter Six, many of these medications can affect your baby if they are present in your body at the time you conceive.

Counter the effects of stress with good nutrition, including the foods, vitamins, and minerals in the Fertility Food Plan in the next chapter. In addition, mild exercise, combined with adequate rest, fresh air, and, when possible, sunshine, can help your body cope with stress.

Finally, try to smile, even when you don't feel like it. The newest studies show that when the muscles of the face form a smile, a biochemical message is relayed to your brain to produce endorphins, powerful body chemicals that can, among other things, help us combat stress and promote fertility!

· 11 ·

THE FERTILITY DIET PROGRAM

The Foods and Vitamins That Can Help You Get Pregnant

While most of the research in the field of nutrition has not been directly in the area of fertility, much of what has been learned generally relates to your reproductive health. Studies show that regardless of your weight, *what* you eat as well as *how much* you eat in the months and weeks prior to getting pregnant are important variables in your fertility equation. Certainly my own patients have proved this time and again. In the past several years many of them have improved the status of their reproductive health through good nutrition, and many even have overcome certain types of infertility simply by changing their eating habits.

HOW FOOD AFFECTS YOUR FERTILITY

Perhaps the most important link between food and fertility is simply eating the right *amount* of food both before and after you get pregnant. If you are not taking in enough calories, you might not get pregnant at all. Recent studies show that when calorie consumption is low, ovulation can come to a complete halt. Often women with anorexia nervosa (an eating disorder) lose their menstrual cycle altogether and have almost no reproductive hormones circulating through their bodies.

Even more important, however, is what can happen if you do get pregnant when calorie intake is insufficient. Research beginning as early as World War II and continuing to the present shows that mothers who restrict their food intake to between 900 and 1200 calories a day in the weeks prior to conception can give birth to children who not only are smaller at birth, but have an infant death rate three times that of women who eat proper amounts of food.

Other new studies have found that continuing to consume insufficient calories after you conceive can cause your baby to suffer intrauterine growth retardation (IUGR), a condition in which there are inadequate food stores for growth. As a result, your baby is at increased risk for premature birth, heart distress, even death. After birth he or she can develop dangerously low glucose and/or calcium levels.

The good news is that by making sure you eat enough both before and after you get pregnant, you can increase your chances for not only a fast conception, but a healthy baby!

ARE YOU EATING ENOUGH TO GET PREGNANT?

According to the most recent U.S. Department of Agriculture (USDA) Nationwide Food Consumption Survey, women are currently consuming 200 calories a day *fewer* than they did fifteen years ago. The study also shows that more than three-quarters of the participants did not meet the basic nutritional requirements for proper body functioning.

The U.S. Department of Health maintains that if you are not underweight or overweight your body needs about 2,100 calories a day to function properly. Just prior to conception that need can rise as high as 2,300 calories a day, while after conception you should be consuming 2,500 to 2,700 calories a day.

WHAT YOU EAT MATTERS, TOO— WHY CALORIES ALONE ARE NOT ENOUGH!

Equally important as getting *enough* food is making certain that you eat the *right* foods—meals that are nutritionally balanced and contain adequate amounts of all the basic vitamins and minerals.

While I have always believed in the power of good nutrition to enhance both a patient's and her partner's fertility, science is now beginning to *prove* that this is so. Recent studies conducted and/or reported by the National Network to Prevent Birth Defects have shown that eating nutritiously can help you counter some of the fertility-robbing effects of many toxic influences like cigarette smoke, alcohol, drugs, birth control pills, and air pollution. Independent studies have shown, moreover, that diets that are nutritionally balanced and meet the minimum daily requirement of vitamins and minerals can also help decrease your risk of pregnancy-related problems like prolonged labor, hypertension, gestational diabetes, preeclampsia, infection, and excessive bleeding.

GOOD NUTRITION IS GOOD FOR YOUR BABY

In addition to helping you, eating nutritiously both before and after you conceive can also help you have a healthier baby. In a recent study of 23,000 women conducted at the Boston University Center for Human Genetics it was learned that by simply meeting a daily dietary requirement of 1 milligram (mg) of folic acid (a derivative of vitamin C) in the first six weeks of your pregnancy, you can decrease your baby's risk of neural tube defect (a serious congenital malformation that can result in infant death) to one-quarter that of the average. Studies currently in progress promise to link even more fertility-related consequences to vitamin and mineral deficiencies.

Since you may be pregnant six, eight, or even ten weeks before knowing it, building adequate prepregnancy nutritional reserves can help ensure that your body will always be ready to protect your baby, regardless of when your conception occurs!

THE FERTILITY POWER BOOST: WHAT TO EAT TO GET PREGNANT

Later in this chapter you will find my Fertility Food Plan, the diet program I developed to help my patients meet the nutritional and caloric demands of conception and pregnancy. However, you can make any eating plan more nutritionally sound if you follow these guidelines in each of your meals:

- Carbohydrates: 45 to 55 percent[1]
  (about 1,200 to 1,400 calories daily)
- Protein: 12 to 14 percent[1]
  (about 45 to 50 grams, or 200 calories daily)
- Fats: 30 percent or less[2]
  (about 50 to 60 grams, or 500 calories daily)
- Sodium: 1,000 to 3,300 mg daily[3]
- Cholesterol: 300 mg daily[2]

In addition, I have found that many of my patients were able to have a fast, easy conception when they increased their overall caloric intake by adding 10 to 12 percent more protein (especially lean red meat) to their daily diet in the month prior to when they plan to get pregnant. How can this help? Studies show that meals that are high in protein, especially those containing lean red meat, promote ovulation. Conversely, diets that are deficient in protein can disrupt the menstrual cycle and cause at least

[1] Recommended daily allowance.
[2] American Heart Association.
[3] USDA

a temporary, and sometimes a more long-lasting, bout with infertility. According to the American College of Obstetricians and Gynecologists (ACOG), an adequate amount of protein in your diet (at least 200 calories daily) can increase your developing baby's birthweight and may protect you from premature delivery.

Finally, I have also found that having my patients eat more *complex* carbohydrates (like whole grain breads, fruits, vegetables, and pasta), as opposed to *simple* carbohydrates (like white bread, cake, and sugary snacks) can improve fertility as well. Studies show that complex carbohydrates promote the functioning of your body's neurotransmitters, the biochemical messengers that carry hormonal signals and other important reproductive data from your brain to your body.

Most important, remember that nutrition is an *interdependent concept*. Each food you eat *needs* components of other foods in order to be of maximum value. When your diet is balanced, all the calories you consume are supereffective. Without this nutritional *teamwork,* depletions capable of harming your fertility can eventually develop.

DO HEALTH FOODS MAKE A HEALTHIER BABY?

Although studies confirming a decision either way are scarce, it is my personal belief that the fewer chemicals, toxins, and pollutants you put in your system around the time of conception and certainly after you are pregnant, the healthier your baby will be.

THE BAD-NEWS FOODS: WHAT TO AVOID IF YOU WANT TO CONCEIVE

In addition to the ways in which *good foods* encourage your fertility, there are some bad-news foods which, because of harmful ingredients or their ability to rob key nutrients from your body, can work against your reproductive health and may even interfere with your ability to get pregnant. Some, when eaten on a regular basis, can cause you or your baby real harm.

What should you avoid when trying to conceive? Although in many cases reports are still inconclusive, I advise my patients against the following:

- ◆ Artificial sweeteners, particularly saccharin, which, according to studies presented at a recent meeting of the American College of Nutrition, may not be safe to consume either prior to conception or after you are pregnant. Studies on aspartame and other new sweeteners are still being conducted, but it is my personal suggestion that you avoid these products as well until reports are conclusive.
- ◆ Soda, high-sugar fruit drinks, and candy, because excessive sugar can

exacerbate hypoglycemia (a lowering of blood sugar), which in turn can upset levels of reproductive hormones.

- ◆ Peanut butter and spinach, because they can cause a calcium deficiency. According to Cedric Garland, Ph.D., director of the epidemiology program of the Cancer Center at the University of California at San Diego, the latest research shows that these foods, along with those high in sugar, can cause potentially dangerous calcium depletions.
- ◆ *Rare* red meat, because of its link to toxoplasmosis (see Chapter Twelve), a virus that often resides in undercooked meats and can cause birth defects.
- ◆ Frankfurters, bologna, salami, and other lunch meats, because they contain nitrates and nitrites, which can exacerbate the growth of some reproductive cancers.

Finally, while it's important to include *some* fat in your diet, meals that are high in saturated fats (especially dishes that are fried or contain large amounts of tropical oils, such as palm or coconut oil, or lard) should be avoided.

In addition to basic health concerns (like the suspected link between fatty foods and heart disease), excessive dietary fat has also been linked to estrogen overloads, which in turn can exacerbate conditions like endometriosis and some forms of breast disease, including breast cancer.

CAFFEINE AND YOUR FERTILITY: THE IMPORTANT NEW LINK

One of the most important new findings to recently emerge is the correlation between the ability to get pregnant and the consumption of caffeine. Caffeine is believed to interfere with the functioning of the hypothalamus, and ultimately cause ovulation problems, new studies by the National Institutes of Health reveal that ingesting the amount of caffeine found in just one five-ounce cup of coffee (115 mg) you are half as likely to become pregnant as women who drink less than one cup per day.

Although the effects of caffeine on fertility generally disappear once consumption is decreased or eliminated, still research indicates the less you consume, the better your chances of getting pregnant. For this reason, I advise all my fertility patients to avoid the following:

- ◆ Tea: one five-ounce cup contains about 40 to 60 mg of caffeine.
- ◆ Coffee: one five-ounce cup contains from 105 to 115 mg of caffeine.
- ◆ Cola: one twelve-ounce glass has 30 to 40 mg of caffeine.
- ◆ Chocolate: each ounce has about 5 to 10 mg of caffeine.
- ◆ Cocoa: each five-ounce cup has about 4 mg of caffeine.

In addition, many pain relievers also contain significant amounts of caffeine, ranging from 30 mg per tablet up, including:

- Excedrin Extra Strength
- Maximum Strength Midol
- Vanquish
- Anacin
- Amaphen

Finally, note that many over-the-counter diet pills like Dexatrim and stimulants like No-Doz and Efed II also contain anywhere from 100 to 200 mg of caffeine per pill, as do many diuretics. Also check the ingredients of cough medicines, over-the-counter cold medicines, and especially allergy pills; they may contain 16 mg of caffeine per tablet, or more.

VEGETARIAN DIETS AND FERTILITY

If you are currently on a vegetarian diet, careful meal planning is necessary if you are to conceive and deliver a healthy child. Often vegetarian diets are low in calories and sometimes deficient in complete proteins, both of which can lower conception odds. In addition, *strict* vegetarian diets can sometimes lack four important fertility nutrients normally found in meat, fish, and poultry: zinc, vitamin B_{12}, iron, and folic acid.

To make your vegetarian diet work for your fertility and not against it, take nutritional supplements. In addition both you *and* your doctor must remain on the lookout for any signs of nutritional depletion, such as iron deficiency anemia, or other symptoms of vitamin shortages. Also be certain that your percentage of body fat does not drop too low.

In addition, make a special effort to raise the protein levels of the food you eat by mixing and matching, in as many meals as possible, complementary food sources to form a *complete* balance such as:

- Legumes and grains
- Legumes and nuts
- Grains and dairy foods

Finally, you should simply eat more food, more often. By increasing your intake of complex carbohydrates and grains, you can add substantial calories to your daily diet. Eating six or seven smaller meals a day can help you take in more calories than if you try to eat three large meals.

WHAT'S YOUR FOOD I.Q.?

Living in the weight-conscious, diet-crazed world that we do, it's sometimes easier than we realize to become undernourished. Although your weight is a good barometer of whether or not you are taking in enough calories (see the fertility height and weight chart in Chapter Nine), calorie counting alone is often not enough to ensure that all your needs are met. To discover if you are undernourished right now, answer *yes* or *no* to the following questions.

1. Do you eat at least 45 grams (180 calories) of protein a day?
2. Do you eat two servings of vegetables per day?
3. Are you a nonsmoker, and do you drink alcohol very rarely?
4. Do you take a prenatal or superhigh-potency vitamin every day?
5. Do you eat two pieces of fresh fruit every day?
6. Do you eat at least four foods a day high in calcium?
7. Have you not taken birth control pills for at least three months?
8. Do you rarely eat processed foods or frozen dinners?

If you answered *no* to even *one* of the above eight questions, you could be lacking an important nutrient. If you answered *no* to three or more, it's possible you may have some severe nutritional depletions.

FERTILITY VITAMINS: THE SUPPLEMENTS THAT CAN HELP YOU GET PREGNANT

Unfortunately, even a diet that is scrupulously planned may not provide you with all the nutrients you need to protect your fertility—and your baby. Food processing, along with environmental and lifestyle factors, can rob the nutrients you take in, allowing even the most nutritious pre- and postconception diet to come up dangerously short. This is where vitamin and mineral *supplements* can help.

Most fertility specialists now agree that the best way to ensure that you are meeting the minimum daily vitamin and mineral requirements necessary for optimum fertility is to take one to two prenatal vitamins a day (the kind normally taken by women already pregnant), starting six months prior to when you want to conceive. Sold under brand names like Stuart Natal One Plus One, Natabec Rx, and Natalins Rx, these vitamins are available by prescription only. If your doctor does not automatically recommend prenatal vitamins, do bring them to his or her attention.

WHEN MORE SUPPLEMENTS ARE NEEDED: HOW TO TELL

Although prenatal vitamins *are* a good beginning, no one vitamin supplement can guarantee everyone peak nutritional status. Studies show that even when basic vitamin requirements are met, there are still some factors that routinely cause depletions. Many can affect fertility.

If you are planning to get pregnant and any of the following factors are present in your life, you may need to increase your nutrient intake over and above what your prenatal vitamin provides.

You may need supplements if:

- Your regular diet has consisted primarily of carbohydrates, processed sugars, and artificially sweetened foods.
- You eat a lot of chocolate, drink coffee, tea, or colas.
- You regularly use recreational drugs.
- You smoke more than ten cigarettes a day.
- You consume more than two alcoholic drinks a day (or fourteen drinks per week).
- You currently take birth control pills, or took them for a long period of time.
- You live or work in a highly polluted or industrialized area.
- You have fibroid tumors, excessive menstrual bleeding, or anemia.

To find exactly which *extra* supplements you may need, see the Fertility Vitamin and Mineral Support Guide at the end of this chapter.

FERTILITY NUTRIENTS FOR YOUR PARTNER

Although it is *your* body that will conceive and carry a baby, the health of your partner's body also plays a vital role in conception. Nutritional deficiencies in him can adversely affect sperm count and quality. In some

IMPORTANT
WARNING ABOUT
VITAMINS!

Sometimes taking too many vitamins and minerals can be as bad as taking too few, especially after you conceive. Once your pregnancy is confirmed, consult your doctor concerning the exact type of prenatal vitamin (and the amount) you should be taking and whether you will need to add more supplements.

cases, a simple vitamin deficiency could cause sperm count to drop to almost zero! To help protect his fertility, be certain he takes at least one high-potency multivitamin a day. In addition, in the month prior to conceiving he should consult his physician about fortifying his multivitamin with additional supplements until the following *maximum daily totals* are met:

Vitamin A: 10,000 IU daily
Vitamin D: 400 mg daily
Vitamin E: 800 IU daily
Vitamin C: 1,500 mg daily
Vitamin B complex: 100 mg daily
Vitamin B_6: 500 mg total daily, balanced with the 100 mg B complex
Calcium: 800 mg daily
Zinc: 100 mg daily

A FOOD STRATEGY FOR GETTING PREGNANT

Based on guidelines for perinatal care set down by the American College of Obstetricians and Gynecologists, as well as many years of personal experience involving thousands of my own patients, I have devised a Fertility Food Plan, a diet that has helped many of my patients enhance their fertility and give birth to healthier babies overall. Some of my patients who previously suffered from unexplained infertility were able to conceive within just six months of following this food plan and taking vitamin supplements.

Unlike other diets that utilize specific recipes and rigid structured meals, the Fertility Food Plan offers great freedom of personal choice. Assuming that you have already achieved your proper preconception weight (see Chapter Nine), this diet has only two requirements:

1. You must choose the recommended number of servings from each food group *every day*.
2. Your food intake goal must be 2,100 to 2,300 calories per day.

As long as you meet these requisites, you can personalize this diet in any way that suits your appetite and your life-style.

* You can eat any of the foods in any of the groups at any time of the day, and you can vary your meals according to your appetite and your lifestyle. One day you can have a large breakfast, a small lunch, and a medium dinner; at another time you can eat lightly in the morning and have a heavier meal at midday or at night.
* You can split your meals any way you like, eating as often as you like,

as long as you remain within the calorie count. As mentioned, I advocate six or seven small meals, rather than three large ones, to help keep blood sugar at a stable level. Studies show this may have beneficial effects on reproductive hormones, as well as alleviating some of the symptoms of PMS.

♦ You can also use any healthful recipes you like in preparing your meals. For variety, try combining ingredients from more than one food group in one dish, like pasta with vegetables or macaroni and cheese. Or combine different items in one food group, for example, in fruit salad or in a health salad. Use your imagination and feel free to experiment!

THE FERTILITY FOOD PLAN
CALORIC GOAL: 2,100–2,300 PER DAY

Choose the recommended servings from each of the following six food groups:

GROUP 1: MEAT, FISH, POULTRY, AND BEANS

These foods ensure adequate protein intake, as well as providing iron and other essential vitamins.

Recommended Amount:
Three 3- to 4-ounce servings per day

Average Number of Calories per Day:
600

Suggested Sources:

- ♦ White meat chicken, no skin
- ♦ White meat turkey, no skin
- ♦ Turkey leg, no skin
- ♦ Veal—any style
- ♦ Lean beef—any style
- ♦ Tuna—packed in water
- ♦ Dry beans, lentils and other legumes

In addition, you can have any type of broiled or baked fish, including flounder, cod, sole, shrimp, scallops, or lobster. You should also include a portion of any type of liver in your diet at least once a week, broiled or baked.

Two eggs (cooked well to avoid bacterial infections—hard boiled being the best way) can be eaten up to three times weekly.

GROUP 2: COMPLEX CARBOHYDRATES AND GRAINS

These foods provide energy, and studies show they may help encourage the flow of reproductive hormones by promoting better functioning of brain-to-body signals. They also provide important vitamins and minerals.

Recommended Amount:
Five or more 1-cup servings per day

Average Number of Calories per Day:
600 to 800

Suggested Sources:

- ◆ Whole-grain pasta
- ◆ Potato (one medium baked)
- ◆ Rice
- ◆ Oatmeal
- ◆ Cereal (dry), 1 ounce
- ◆ Oat, wheat, or bran muffins (one average muffin equals one serving)
- ◆ Whole wheat bread (one slice equals one serving)

GROUP 3: CALCIUM

These foods provide not only calcium, but phosphorus, protein, and important vitamins necessary for the healthy functioning of your reproductive system.

Recommended Amount:
Four or more servings

Average Number of Calories per Day:
400 to 500

Average Serving Size:
One cup (or equivalent)

Suggested Sources:

- ◆ Low-fat milk (one 8-ounce glass)
- ◆ Low-fat yogurt (12 ounces)
- ◆ Low-fat cottage cheese (1⅓ cups)
- ◆ Cheese (1½ ounces, or 1½ slices)
- ◆ Broccoli (1 cup)

- Sardines (3 ounces)
- Kale (1 cup)
- Low-fat ice cream (1½ cups)

GROUP 4: FRUITS AND VEGETABLES

These foods help you fight off infections that can disrupt fertility, in addition to providing vitamins and minerals. Select one serving rich in vitamin A (a dark yellow or leafy green vegetable) and one serving rich in vitamin C (for example, a citrus fruit). Opt for fresh produce, and eat it raw or lightly steamed.

Recommended Amount:
Four or more servings per day

Average Number of Calories per Day:
300 to 400

Serving Size:
Vegetables: 1 cup raw, ½ cup cooked
Fruit: 1 medium-size fruit, ½ cup fruit juice, ½ cup cooked fruit

Suggested Sources:

VEGETABLES:	FRUITS:
• Cabbage	• Oranges
• Brussels sprouts	• Grapefruits (one-half per serving)
• Carrots	• Apples
• Green beans	• Bananas
• Broccoli	• Cantaloupes (one-half per serving)
• Winter squash	• Honeydew melon (one-half per serving)
• Cauliflower	• Strawberries (½ cup per serving)

GROUP 5: LIQUIDS

Recommended Amount
Eight to ten cups daily (including milk and fruit juices)

Choose from the Following:

- Spring water
- Tap water
- Low-sodium bouillon
- Herbal tea

- ◆ Seltzer (plain or flavored)
- ◆ Low-sodium clear soup

GROUP 6: FATS

Recommended Amount:
About 2 teaspoons daily

Average Number of Calories per Day:
100 maximum

Choose from the Following:

- ◆ Butter
- ◆ Margarine
- ◆ Polyunsaturated oil
- ◆ Low-sodium salad dressing

SAMPLE MENU PLAN FOR ONE DAY

Meal 1:
Orange juice (1 cup) (group 4)
Toast (two slices) (group 2)
Milk (8 oz.) (group 3)
Eggs (two) (group 1)

Meal 2:
Cantaloupe (one-half) (group 4)
Veal patty with cheese on whole wheat toast (groups 1, 2, 3)
Lettuce-and-tomato salad (group 4), with cold-pressed sesame seed oil
  and vinegar dressing (group 6)
Spring water (8 oz.)

Meal 3:
Broccoli (1 cup) (group 4)
Pasta (1 cup) (group 2)
Milk (8 oz.) (group 3)
White meat turkey (3–4 oz.) (group 1)
Apple (one) (group 4)

Meal 4:
Bran muffin (one) (group 2)
Milk (8 oz.) (group 3)

Meal 5:
Yogurt (12 oz.) (group 3)
Vegetable juice (1 cup) (group 4)
Whole wheat crackers (four) (group 2)

Meal 6:
Ice cream (1½ cups) (group 3)
Spring water (8 oz.)

Add one to two glasses of spring water, herbal tea, or bouillon between meals.

THE FERTILITY VITAMIN–MINERAL SUPPORT GUIDE

NUTRIENT: VITAMIN A

ACOG Recommendations:
Up to 100 micrograms retinol equivalents daily

Effects on Fertility:
Although studies linking vitamin A to fertility are scarce, there is evidence that in some women, deficiencies can contribute to symptoms of PMS by affecting levels of estrogen and progesterone. Since these same imbalances can also contribute to biochemical infertility, researchers theorize that vitamin A deficiencies may, in some women, also be linked to infertility.

Because vitamin A is essential to sperm production, deficiencies in men have been directly linked to infertility. Although treatment with vitamin A will not improve the fertility status of men who have no deficiencies, if a lack of this vitamin does exist, supplements can restore sperm count and improve potency.

Role in Pregnancy:
Forms baby's tooth enamel and hair, helps growth of thyroid gland

Signs of Depletion:
Night blindness, rough, dry skin, decreased sense of smell, fatigue, skin blemishes

My Recommended Supplements:
Men: Up to 10,000 IUs daily
Women: None. Take only what is present in prenatal vitamin. An excess of vitamin A can lead to increased risk of birth defects.

NUTRIENT: VITAMIN B_1

ACOG Recommendations:
1.1 mg daily

Effects on Fertility:
No information available

Role in Pregnancy:
Aids in baby's growth and development, contributes to successful breast-feeding

Signs of Depletion:
Easy fatigue, loss of appetite, irritability, emotional instability

My Suggested Supplements:
Men and Women:
100 mg B-complex supplement

NUTRIENT: VITAMIN B_2

ACOG Recommendations:
1.2 to 1.5 mg daily

Effects on Fertility:
No information available

Role in Pregnancy:
Aids in general growth and development of fetus. Deficiencies in mother during pregnancy linked to cleft palate, heart malformations, lack of growth of arm and leg bones, eye problems

Signs of Depletion:
Sore mouth, including cracks in lips, red, sore tongue, visual disturbances, eye fatigue, scaly skin, dizziness

My Suggested Supplement:
Men and Women: 100 mg B complex daily

NUTRIENT: VITAMIN B_3

ACOG Recommendation:
13 to 16 mg daily

Effects on Fertility:
Because niacin is necessary for the synthesis of the sex hormones needed for conception, researchers theorize that fertility will suffer if this nutrient is in short supply.

Role in Pregnancy:
Builds brain cells and transfers energy to your baby

Signs of Depletion:
Muscular weakness, general fatigue, loss of appetite, indigestion, bad breath, insomnia, depression

My Suggested Supplements:
Men and Women: 100 mg B complex daily

NUTRIENT: VITAMIN B_6

ACOG Recommendation:
2 to 2.5 mg daily

Effects on Fertility:
Some reports have indicated that vitamin B_6 may increase fertility by increasing levels of serotonin and dopamine, two brain chemicals that influence the production of the reproductive hormones FSH and LH, the biochemicals necessary for egg production and release. When levels are low, some studies have indicated that these reproductive hormones may end up in short supply.

Because it helps regulate the menstrual cycle, B_6 may also encourage fertility by promoting a more regular ovulation.

Finally, preliminary reports made as early as 1979 showed that unexplained infertility could be overcome when women were given between 100 and 800 mg of B_6 daily. Because the sample studied was small, the results are not considered conclusive. However, they do indicate that B_6 has at least some influence on your reproductive system.

Role in Pregnancy:
Aids in development of healthy fetus. Helps ease morning sickness during first trimester of pregnancy. Deficiency during pregnancy can lead to edema (swelling) and high blood pressure, as well as to increased risk of cleft palate in your baby.

Signs of Depletion:
Depression, dermatitis

My Suggested Supplements:
Men and Women: Up to 500 mg daily, in balance with 100 mg B complex. Stop supplements and rely only on prenatal vitamins after pregnancy has been confirmed.

NUTRIENT: VITAMIN B_{12}

ACOG Recommendation:
3 to 4 mg daily

Effects on Fertility:
Because studies show a deficiency can exacerbate menstrual disturbances, including irregular cycles, researchers believe a link may exist between B_{12} and fertility. Although studies are scarce, some preliminary work indicates the connecting factor may be the influence of B_{12} on regular ovulation.

Role in Pregnancy:
Aids in development of baby's red blood cells, helps avoid oxygen deprivation, which can lead to birth defects, especially brain damage

Signs of Depletion:
Nervousness, body odor, menstrual disturbances, difficulty in walking

My Suggested Supplements:
Men and Women: 100 mg B complex daily

NUTRIENT: VITAMIN C

ACOG Recommendations:
60 mg daily before pregnancy, 80 mg daily after conception

Effects on Fertility:
As we age, our sex glands develop a greater need for vitamin C and will draw it from other tissues if supplies are limited. Once those sources have been depleted, these glands can become severely impaired, often affecting your ability to reproduce.

Conversely, when vitamin C intake is too high, it can also increase your risk of reproductive problems, including infertility, premature birth, and miscarriage.

In men, a number of studies have linked deficiencies to poor sperm motility, viability, and maturity and to inadequate percentages of perfect sperm. In some men with severe deficiencies, one 500-mg vitamin C tablet taken every twelve hours has restored fertility in just four days.

Finally, studies at the University of Texas Medical Branch in Galveston found that vitamin C may hasten the elimination from the body of lead, nicotine, and other toxic substances capable of harming fertility.

Role in Pregnancy:
Aids in development of baby's skin, tendons, and bones through the formation of collagen. Maternal deficiencies can cause abnormalities in baby's bones and teeth.

Signs of Depletion:
Shortness of breath, impaired digestion, bleeding gums, tendency to bruise, slow healing of wounds

My Suggested Supplements:
Men: Up to 1,500 mg daily
Women: Up to 1,000 mg daily over what a prenatal vitamin offers until pregnancy is confirmed, after which time one to two prenatal vitamins daily supply all your basic needs. Important: depleting factors include aspirin, birth control pills, stress, tobacco, alcohol, and recreational drugs.

NUTRIENT: FOLIC ACID

ACOG Recommendations:
400 mg daily before conception
Up to 800 mg daily after conception

Effects on Fertility:
Because a folic acid deficiency has been linked to anemia, studies indicate this nutrient may influence fertility by affecting the energy levels necessary for proper functioning of the pituitary and hypothalamus glands, two major sources of important fertility hormones. In addition, a folic acid deficiency before and after conception can increase your risk of birth defects, premature birth, and miscarriage.

Role in Pregnancy:
Aids in manufacture of cells and in overall development of baby. Deficiencies in mother prior to pregnancy linked to increased risk of cleft palate, brain damage, poor learning skills, and neural tube defects in baby. In pregnancy, deficiencies can lead to toxemia.

Signs of Depletion:
Prematurely gray hair, inflamed tongue, gastrointestinal disturbances, anemia

My Suggested Supplements:
Men: None. A multivitamin containing folic acid meets requirements.
Women: Up to 1 mg daily, including amount in prenatal vitamin

NUTRIENT: VITAMIN D

ACOG Recommendations:
10 to 15 micrograms daily

Effects on Fertility
Because some vitamin D receptors are found in the hypothalamus gland and in the ovaries, deficiencies might impair reproductive functions, both in men and in women. (See Chapter Thirteen, "How the Sun Can Help You Get Pregnant.")

Role in Pregnancy:
Builds calcium into bones and teeth of developing baby

Signs of Depletion:
Tetany, a muscular weakness, with numbness, tingling, and muscle spasms

My Suggested Supplements:
Men: Up to 400 mg daily
Women: Only that present in one to two prenatal vitamins daily. Excess vitamin D during the first twelve weeks of pregnancy has been linked to birth defects.

For Your Information:
A fat-soluble vitamin that is not readily excreted, vitamin D is now added to many foods, so supplements are rarely necessary. It is also made naturally by your body when you are exposed to the sun, although all production stops when you get a suntan. Because pregnancy can make some women highly sensitive to vitamin D, toxic levels (especially those linked to birth defects) can occur if you take as little as two to three times the recommended daily allowance.

NUTRIENT: VITAMIN E

ACOG Recommendation:
Up to 10 mg daily

Effects on Fertility:
A number of studies have shown that severe vitamin E deficiencies may be linked to increased risk of premature labor and/or miscarriage. In addition, research has found that vitamin E helps to regulate the menstrual flow, by cutting back on excessive blood loss or increasing scanty bleeding, depending on your needs. It can also have a positive effect on the menstrual rhythm, leading some researchers to believe it may increase fertility by helping to regulate ovulation.

Studies involving male fertility and vitamin E have shown that deficiencies may lead to degeneration of testicle tissue, affecting sperm production and maturation. Once this type of damage occurs, restoring deficiencies won't help, so it's essential that your partner never allow even a slight dip in E levels. Important: Although it's stored in the liver, fatty tissue, heart, muscles, testes, uterus, blood, and adrenal and pituitary glands, vitamin E only remains in the body a short time, with 60 to 70 percent excreted in the feces, so a deficiency can easily occur.

Role in Pregnancy:
Promotes lung maturation. When premature births are the result of E deficiencies, infants can be born susceptible to anemia. When the child's E quotient is low, hemorrhaging can occur; the blood cells of E-deficient babies are also prone to weakness.

Signs of Depletion:
Gastrointestinal distress, anemia, rupture of red blood cells

My Suggested Supplements:
Men: Up to 800 IUs daily total
Women: Up to 400 IUs daily, in addition to a prenatal supplement (about 800 IUs daily), until pregnancy is confirmed. Once you are pregnant, stop all supplements; rely only on prenatal vitamins.

THE ESSENTIAL MINERALS

In addition to vitamins, the following four minerals have special importance in relation to fertility and pregnancy:

CALCIUM

ACOG Recommendation:
800 to 1,600 mg daily

Effects on Fertility:
When calcium is in short supply, the output of estrogen decreases. Since

your reproductive health depends not only on the presence of estrogen, but on precise amounts of this hormone (see Chapter Nine), a calcium deficiency can cause estrogen levels to plummet, affecting egg production as well as ovulation.

Role in Pregnancy:
Beginning in the second trimester, calcium is utilized to form your baby's skeletal system and teeth. It is also essential for lactation. A deficiency can cause your baby to develop bones that are less dense and weaker than normal.

Signs of Depletion:
Numbness and tingling in arms and legs, cramps in muscles, joint pains, heart palpitations, slow pulse rates, tooth decay, insomnia, excessive irritability of nerves and muscles, menstrual pain, PMS.

My Suggested Supplements:
Men: Up to 800 mg daily
Women: Up to 500 mg daily, in addition to your prenatal vitamin, depending on depletion factors

IRON

ACOG Recommendation:
18 mg daily before pregnancy
Up to 75 mg daily after pregnancy

Effects on Fertility:
By causing anemia, iron deficiencies can disrupt the menstrual cycle, in some cases bringing it to a complete halt. (Some believe this disruption might be your body's natural defense system for conserving depleted red blood cells.) If your menstrual cycle *is* affected by iron deficiency anemia, the timing and function of ovulation and all reproductive hormones can be thrown out of kilter, leaving fertility to suffer.

Role in Pregnancy:
Needed by your baby to form his or her own blood cells and to build a stored supply. Most fetal iron is obtained through the placental blood flow, but some can be taken directly from your body as well. The fetus, the placenta, and your own expanded blood volume during pregnancy require considerable iron, so supplements are always recommended.

It is extremely vital that you correct all iron deficiencies prior to conceiving, since a depletion that continues could be a sign of anemia. The latest studies show if you are anemic when you conceive, you increase your chances of a premature birth and other pregnancy complications.

Signs of Depletion:
Anemia, pale skin, abnormal fatigue, constipation, lusterless and brittle nails, difficulty in breathing. Calcium and iron are the most commonly deficient nutrients in women. Prior to pregnancy your body absorbs about 10 percent of the iron you take in, but by the time you are into your second trimester, your iron intake increases threefold. (Absorption is also increased by vitamin C, folic acid and B_{12}.)

My Suggested Supplements:
Men: Unless anemia exists, a multivitamin should cover all needs. If signs of depletion exist, see your doctor before taking supplements.
Women: One to two iron pills a day, depending on depletion factors.

MINERAL: MAGNESIUM

ACOG Recommendation:
300 to 450 mg daily, or one-half the amount of calcium supplement

Effects on Fertility:
See Calcium, Effects on Fertility.

Role in Pregnancy:
Allows your baby to absorb adequate calcium for development of bone and teeth

Signs of Depletion:
Apprehension, muscle twitch, tremors, confusion, disorientation

My Suggested Supplements:
Men and Women: One-half the amount of your calcium supplement.

MINERAL: ZINC

ACOG Recommendation:
15 to 20 mg daily

Effects on Fertility:
As early as puberty, deficiencies can cause development problems in your sex organs, inhibiting growth and maturation. Later in life, zinc deficiencies have been associated with various types of reproductive problems.

In men even a minimal zinc deficiency can cause infertility by reducing both testosterone levels and sperm count. It also can lead to unhealthy changes in the size and structure of the prostate gland, which contains more zinc than any other part of the body. In prostate illness, especially cancer, zinc levels drop, leading to infertility.

Role in Pregnancy:
Deficiencies during pregnancy produce a variety of birth defects, including skeletal and brain malformations, cardiovascular problems, and defects in the central nervous system of your baby. A zinc deficiency can also cause you prolonged labor, excess bleeding, eclampsia, higher risk of infection, and hypertension during your pregnancy.

Signs of Depletion:
Abnormal fatigue, loss of normal taste sensitivity, poor appetite, and suboptimal growth

My Suggested Supplements:
Men: Up to 100 mg daily
Women: Up to 20 mg daily, in addition to your prenatal vitamin, depending on depletion factors

MEGADOSING: TOO MUCH OF A GOOD THING?

A number of years ago some researchers began advocating supplement megadosing, the practice of using excessively large amounts of vitamins and minerals (more than ten times the recommended daily allowance per dose) to treat everything from stress to immune system deficiencies to disease—even infertility! Can massive doses of vitamins help—and more important, can they hurt you or your baby? It's easier to develop toxic effects from the fat-soluble vitamins—A, D, and E—because they are stored in your body; the water-soluble vitamins—C and B complex— leave your body within twenty-four hours, so they're safe in all but the most grossly excessive amounts.

While hard evidence linking nutrient megadoses and fertility and/or pregnancy problems is scarce, the following has been reported:

- *Vitamin A:* Taken in excess of 25,000 IU daily during pregnancy can increase your baby's risk of bladder malformation, cleft palate, eye damage, and webbed fingers and toes.
- *Vitamin D:* More than ten times the RDA may decrease sexual desire.
- *Vitamin B$_6$:* 2,000 to 6,000 mg daily may cause nerve damage.
- *Vitamin C:* 12,000 mg or more daily during pregnancy may cause

your baby to be born with an abnormal dependence on this nutrient, leading to a condition called rebound scurvy, which causes irritability, and pain in arms, legs, bones, and muscles. In addition, excessive vitamin C can decrease the absorption of copper, a trace mineral essential to ovulation, and it can cause a false positive in urine and stool tests.

- *Zinc:* An excess of more than 2,000 mg daily can cause gastrointestinal distress and may upset the balance of other important minerals, bringing about deficiencies that can affect fertility and/or the health of your baby.

By sticking to the formulas found in prenatal vitamin prescriptions (and following your physician's advice about supplements), you can be sure you will be giving your body the most positive nutritional power available.

• 12 •

GETTING READY FOR PREGNANCY

What You Must Do Before You Conceive

While it was once believed that obstetrical treatment should begin only *after* a conception is confirmed, today most forward-thinking physicians realize that many problems can be prevented when the same care begins before you get pregnant. Thus the concept of preconception counseling was born, a new form of nurturing care in which you, your partner, and your doctor work together on a program personally tailored to:

- Encourage a quick and easy conception
- Ensure your health and safety during pregnancy
- Decrease your risk of miscarriage
- Help your baby avoid birth defects

Although preparation for these goals ideally starts about six months prior to when you want to conceive, scheduling a preconception exam at any time prior to getting pregnant can offer a multitude of benefits to you and your baby.

HOW PRECONCEPTION COUNSELING WORKS

The basis of preconception counseling is multifaceted. It takes into consideration not just factors affecting *your* reproductive health, but the joint fertility status of you *and* your partner, as well as a host of shared physical, psychological, and social factors capable of affecting your fertility including:

- ◆ Age
- ◆ Nutritional profile
- ◆ General health
- ◆ Occupation
- ◆ Reproductive history
- ◆ Weight
- ◆ Body fitness
- ◆ Family history
- ◆ Life-style

By carefully evaluating information from many areas of your life, your preconception specialist formulates a risk assessment profile of your pregnancy and determines where potential problems might lie. To help accomplish this, your first preconception counseling visit should include detailed health and lifestyle histories of you and your partner. If your gynecologist is also your preconception specialist, much of this information about you is probably already on file. However, it's still a good idea to discuss your medical history with your doctor at this time and to inform him or her of any pertinent factors about your partner as well.

Prepare for your initial visit by writing down key information; then give these notes to your doctor. I have found this to be extremely helpful, especially in getting to know a new patient, and I often refer to these personal notes throughout the course of treatment.

THE PERSONAL FACTS YOUR DOCTOR NEEDS TO KNOW

1. *Your reproductive history.* Because your reproductive *history* can influence the *future* of your fertility, it's important that your doctor have an accurate, detailed account of any conception-related events that might have occurred:

- ◆ Miscarriages—how often, how many, and when
- ◆ Abortions—how often and how many
- ◆ Reproductive surgeries, including laparoscopies, D&C, treatment for ovarian cysts, etc.
- ◆ Your mother took DES no
- ◆ Number of previous pregnancies

Grammy - infant death (1st child)

◆ History of fetal death, neonatal death, infants with birth defects
◆ History of vaginal bleeding
◆ Ectopic pregnancies

In addition, your doctor should know something about your partner's reproductive history, including:

◆ If he has fathered children
◆ If any previous partners had miscarriages
◆ If he has fathered birth-defected children
◆ If his mother took DES

2. *Family history.* We now know that the family history of both parents can influence the outcome of a pregnancy. To help safeguard your baby before birth, your doctor will need to know if any of the following conditions appear in your background and/or your partner's:

◆ High blood pressure *my Dad, my Grandma M.*
◆ Diabetes *Grandma M. (adult onset)*
◆ Birth defects *∅*
◆ Inherited diseases associated with birth defects (e.g., sickle cell anemia, Tay-Sachs disease) *∅*
◆ Mental retardation *∅*
◆ Cystic fibrosis *∅*

3. *Personal medical history.* Because so much of what is happening in your body today is the result of biological conditions and events that occurred in the past, it is important for your doctor to have a personal history of both you and your partner regarding diseases and conditions or infections that could have a residual effect on fertility, including:

◆ STDs (gonorrhea, chlamydia, syphilis, genital herpes)
◆ Infections of the reproductive tract, especially PID
◆ High blood pressure
◆ Diabetes (type, for how long, any treatment received)
◆ Exposure to x-rays (when, what areas of the body)
◆ Heart disease
◆ Exposure to AIDS
◆ Epilepsy
◆ German measles (important for you)
◆ Mumps (important for your partner)
◆ Any medications you or your partner regularly take, including allergy pills or shots, insulin, antacids, etc.

OTHER VITAL INFORMATION YOUR DOCTOR NEEDS TO KNOW

Since your fertility, your pregnancy, and the health of your baby can also be affected by factors outside the realm of personal biology, your doctor should have information about aspects of your life that could influence your reproductive health. This includes where you and your partner live and work, how each of you earns a living and how you spend your leisure time, both together and apart. Your physician needs to know:

- How much alcohol you and your partner regularly consume
- Your eating habits and your partner's, the number of calories consumed daily, vitamin supplements (if any)
- If either of you smokes, and if so, how much
- If either of you has used illegal drugs, and if so, what and when
- If you or your mate work with radiation or are exposed to any toxic chemicals or substances (see Chapters Five and Six)
- If you own a cat (we'll tell you why in a moment)
- If you take birth control pills or have used them in the past, and when you stopped
- If either of you have or have had sexual relations outside your marriage

THE PRECONCEPTION PHYSICAL: WHAT IT MUST INCLUDE

Once your history has been established, your doctor will begin the physical part of your prepregnancy exam. Like the GYN–T.H.E. exam in Chapter Seven, a thorough preconception physical should include the following:

- A pelvic exam
- Blood pressure and weight check
- Cultures for STDs for which you are exhibiting symptoms or believe you have been exposed to
- A Pap smear for cervical abnormalities
- A thyroid function test

Your doctor should also perform a thorough investigation for heart problems and/or symptoms of an undiagnosed cardiac or vascular condition. These must be under good control before you conceive.

If you have a family history of diabetes or if you are exhibiting symptoms of this disease (including weight loss, excessive thirst and/or urination), you should receive a glucose tolerance test.

Finally, you must have a blood test for anemia, a condition that develops when your oxygen-carrying red blood cells decrease due to any number of causes, including poor nutrition, iron deficiency, internal bleeding, severe menstrual bleeding, or bleeding from fibroid tumors. The test is easy, the treatment is simple, and getting anemia under control before conception can prevent a number of serious birth defects.

THE SPECIAL TESTS TO PROTECT YOUR PREGNANCY

In addition to these standard procedures, your preconception checkup should also include some specific viral diagnostic tests that can help you and your baby avoid problems during your pregnancy. In the past, doctors believed viral tests were only important after you conceived, but today, most progressive fertility specialists find distinct advantages in testing before pregnancy.

Among the most important is knowing whether or not you may have had one of these infections in the past, and now possess the protecting antibodies that develop after the virus leaves your body. Since the symptoms of some of these diseases can go undetected, I have often seen patients who were unaware they had previously been infected until their preconception blood tests revealed they possessed the antibodies that would protect them from reinfection. Knowing your antibody status to several key viruses prior to conceiving can help you to know what extra precautions you must take during your pregnancy to protect your baby from harm.

THE VIRAL TESTS YOU NEED RIGHT NOW!

The TORCH Diseases
(Toxoplasmosis, Rubella, Cytomegalovirus, and Herpes)

TORCH is a relatively new term coined from the names of four major infections that, when contracted during pregnancy, can affect the health of your unborn baby and increase his or her chances for a number of serious birth defects.

TOXOPLASMOSIS
This is an infection that occurs when a parasite found in the intestines of cats, sheep, cattle, and pigs makes its way into your body when you eat meat that is undercooked, or when you come into contact with the feces

of an infected animal. For example, this can happen when you are emptying your cat's litter box or when you are working in the garden, where contaminated stools may have been deposited. Toxoplasmosis is most dangerous in the first trimester of pregnancy, when the virus can attack the fetus and cause a number of serious birth defects.

In adults and children the symptoms of toxoplasmosis can often be so mild that the virus can go completely unnoticed. If your preconception test shows that you do not possess toxoplasmosis antibodies, watch diligently for these symptoms and report them to your doctor immediately:

- ◆ Fever
- ◆ Slight rash
- ◆ General flulike feeling

There is no treatment for toxoplasmosis, but if you contract this virus during your pregnancy, your baby must receive immediate medical attention directly after birth. The most common therapy is folic acid and sulfur and occasionally corticosteroids. While the effects of the virus cannot be reversed, additional problems can sometimes be prevented with immediate medical care.

There is no vaccine for toxoplasmosis, but you can avoid the disease both before and after conception:

- ◆ Make sure all red meat and pork is cooked thoroughly (well-done is best)
- ◆ Avoid cat litter boxes
- ◆ Wear heavy protective gloves when working in the garden

RUBELLA (German measles)

In addition to causing a number of serious birth defects, when contracted during pregnancy, rubella is also one of the most common causes of miscarriage and infant death. Fortunately, if you have had this virus in the past, it is almost impossible for you to be reinfected, so your baby is probably safe. If you have not had rubella, there is a highly effective vaccine capable of protecting you and your unborn child.

If your prepregnancy test shows that you have no rubella antibodies (indicating you have not had this virus), you should be vaccinated prior to conceiving. However, because the rubella vaccine is *live,* you must wait a minimum of three months after receiving it before attempting conception.

Should any of the symptoms of rubella appear during your pregnancy (including a flat red skin rash and a slight fever), see your doctor immediately.

CYTOMEGALOVIRUS

A parasite thought to live silently in the bodies of up to 80 percent of the population, this virus is passed via intimate contact with an infected person. It is usually found in body secretions, such as breast milk, saliva, semen, cervical mucus, urine, and transfused blood, and it is most often transmitted from children to adults who care for them, in day care centers, schools, or especially hospitals.

For the most part, this virus remains dormant until stress, a lowered immune system, or some unknown factor triggers it into activity. If it becomes activated during your pregnancy, birth defects or miscarriage can result.

A most deceiving aspect of cytomegalovirus is that it is usually asymptomatic, so you probably won't know it is residing in your body unless you are tested. When symptoms do appear, they usually resemble a flu, including fever and general aches and pains. There is currently no treatment available, but since the disease usually attacks only those women who are in poor health and/or under prolonged stress, you can protect yourself by getting adequate rest, eating nutritiously, and taking vitamin supplements to support your immune system. In addition, if you do work with children, especially if you are in the health care industry, be certain to wash your hands frequently and give special attention to personal hygiene on the job.

HERPES

Although an outbreak during your pregnancy won't affect your baby, should you have a herpes attack just prior to going into labor, your child could be contaminated during the birthing process. Up to 25 percent of all babies born with herpes can die, and many more can be blinded for life when the virus attacks their eyes.

Since the initial outbreak is always much more severe (and usually lasts longer) than any subsequent reinfections, your doctor needs to know prior to your pregnancy if herpes is present in your system. Should you have an outbreak when you are ready to deliver, a cesarean section will minimize the threat of contamination to your baby.

The treatment regimen for herpes is given in Chapter Four.

The Hepatitis Virus

When contracted during pregnancy, this virus generally does not cause birth defects, but it can do devastating, sometimes permanent, damage to your liver. In addition, it can make your gestational time uncomfortable and uneasy. Moreover, your baby's immune system does not fully develop until after birth, so if this virus is contracted during any stage of your pregnancy, it can easily be passed to your developing fetus, causing weakness and, in rare cases, even death.

Preconception testing for the presence of hepatitis antibodies is most important because the virus can be easily confused with other conditions that can occur during pregnancy, such as mononucleosis, a drug allergy, or a mild jaundice that develops when the weight of your baby presses on your gallbladder and creates a pool of bile in your liver. Symptoms of hepatitis include fatigue, lethargy, nausea, vomiting, and jaundice.

A protective vaccine may be advisable if you are in a high-risk profession: doctor, nurse, dentist, or other medical worker.

THE PRECONCEPTION BLOOD TEST THAT PROTECTS YOUR BABY

In addition to testing for diseases, it's also important that your doctor have on file—and that you know as well—not only your blood type (A, B, or O), but whether you have the Rhesus (Rh) factor, a substance that is found on the surface of red blood cells in the majority of the population.

- If you have the Rh factor, your blood type carries the suffix "positive," as in A-, B-, or O-positive blood.
- If the Rh factor is missing, as it is in 15 to 20 percent of the population, your blood type carries the suffix "negative," as in A-, B-, or O-negative blood.

Whether negative or positive, the Rh factor has no influence on *your* health. However, if your blood is Rh negative, pregnancy-related problems can occur.

How Your Blood Type Can Affect Your Baby

Although for most Rh-negative mothers pregnancy is healthy and normal, problems can develop if your partner's blood is Rh positive. In such a case, your baby's blood can be Rh positive. If, during the course of pregnancy, your baby's Rh-positive blood makes its way into your Rh-negative system (as can happen, for example, during amniocentesis, a test often given to pregnant women over age thirty-five, or during your seventh month of pregnancy, when spontaneous bleeding sometimes occurs), your body will react as it would if your system were invaded by a virus or bacteria: it will create antibodies. Should those antibodies be transferred back into your baby's bloodstream, they will begin destroying your baby's blood. The result is a severe type of anemia known as Rhesus disease. If the disease is left undiagnosed, severe birth defects and/or fetal death can occur. Deprived of precious oxygen-carrying red blood cells, your baby's brain and body literally starve to death.

How to Protect Your Baby Right Now!

The good news is that because the effects of Rh antibodies are cumulative (building in your system each time your body is infused with positive blood), there is very little risk that your first Rh-positive conception will be affected. In fact, most of the time serious problems don't set in until after the second or third Rh-positive pregnancy. And today, even those pregnancies can be protected, thanks to the discovery of the Rhogam injection, a treatment that absorbs any Rh-positive blood cells that enter an Rh-negative system, cutting off the body's need to manufacture antibodies. To be effective, Rhogam must be administered within three days following any event that could allow the passage of Rh-positive blood cells into your body:

- The delivery of an Rh-positive baby
- Amniocentesis of an Rh-positive baby
- Miscarriage or abortion in which the blood type of your baby was unknown
- A stillbirth of an Rh-positive baby
- An ectopic pregnancy

If you are Rh negative and fall into any of the above categories and have not been given Rhogam injections, make your doctor aware of this during your preconception interview.

Once you are pregnant, be certain to be checked frequently for rising levels of antibodies, and receive a Rhogam injection in your seventh month. This should be done even if you don't know your baby's Rh factor.

TESTING FOR GENETIC DISEASES

Although everyone carries four to six genes that have the potential to cause birth defects, most often they remain harmless. However, if you and your partner both carry the same defective gene, your child is at increased risk. Currently, we can identify some 250 genetic defects, but except under extraordinary circumstances, such as a history of genetic diseases in both partners' families, preconception testing should be limited.

Because certain genetic diseases occur more regularly in certain groups, if you and your partner fall into any of the following categories your preconception exam should include blood tests for their related conditions:

- Asian and Mediterranean: test for Thalassemia major (also known as Cooley's anemia)
- Black: test for sickle cell anemia, Cooley's anemia
- Jewish: test for Tay–Sachs disease

In addition, I often suggest genetic testing if my patient and her partner have any of the following factors in their family histories:

◆ Mental retardation
◆ Intellectual impairment
◆ Physical deformities present from birth
◆ Physical disabilities present from birth

Get Tested—But Don't Panic

In gene-related birth defects, both parents must carry the recessive gene in order for the child to be affected. Even then the odds of problems occurring can range from as high as one in two to as low as one in ten thousand or more. For this reason, even a positive genetic test does not mean that your baby will be born defective.

If, however, your preconception tests or your family histories indicate the possibility of a problem, I suggest you seek sophisticated analysis at a genetic counseling center. These are specially equipped laboratories staffed with medical personnel who specialize in gene-related disorders. They can perform special blood tests and provide other background screening prior to conception, as well as fetal tissue and fluid sampling, as early as nine weeks after conception, to help detect any possibility of genetic disorder. If a problem is found, specially trained counselors can review all possible threats to your baby and, if necessary, assist you in exploring alternative ways to achieve parenthood.

TAKE CHARGE OF YOUR PREGNANCY!

Although sometimes it may seem as if there are more chances of things going wrong with a pregnancy than going right, I can promise you that this is not the case. And the concept of preconception counseling is not suggested to frighten you into believing that every pregnancy requires specialized care. In fact, if you are young, and both you and your partner are basically healthy, you probably won't have any problems conceiving *or* delivering a perfect baby on your own.

However, there are factors in today's world, and even in your personal lives, that *can* sometimes act as an obstacle to getting pregnant, making conception and even delivery more difficult than it has to be.

By giving you the opportunity to overcome these obstacles, *before* they have the chance to present problems, preconception counseling offers you an *extra* measure of protection and safety, and a new kind of *complete* control over your childbearing options.

A FINAL WORD:
FINDING A PRECONCEPTION SPECIALIST

Because preconception counseling is still relatively new, not all doctors have incorporated it into their practice. If your gynecologist does not offer this vital service, ask your family doctor to recommend one who does, or check the following resources:

- ◆ *Nearby universities.* Many are affiliated with teaching hospitals and are an excellent source of medical personnel.
- ◆ *Your local hospital.* Call or write to the department of obstetrics, requesting names of physicians who incorporate preconception counseling into their practice.

Finally, don't be afraid to ask an obstetrician who is respected in your community, if he/she offers preconception counseling. If more doctors are aware of the type of care that is important to patients, more may begin to make it available.

· 13 ·

HOW TO GET PREGNANT FAST!

- ◆ Do you make love with the lights on . . . or in the dark?
- ◆ What position do you most often use when making love?
- ◆ What do you do right *before* you have sex . . . and what do you do right afterward?
- ◆ When do you make love—and how often do you have an orgasm?

Although nature plays an important role in getting pregnant, there are many practical aspects of making love that can influence how quickly and easily you conceive. Later in this chapter I will share with you some of the latest findings and pass along helpful suggestions from my own patients.

However, the first and most important way to ensure that you will get pregnant right away is to make love as close to the time of ovulation as possible. Why is this important? Because virtually from the moment your egg is released, it begins to age. In fact, once ovulated, your egg remains fertile for just twenty-four hours. After that it begins to disintegrate. For some women it remains fresh enough for optimum fertilization for only six to eight hours after release.

Although this window of fertilization opportunity is very confined, nature has provided for its limitations by allowing sperm to live in the body for up to two days after it has been ejaculated. (This is why you are considered fertile for up to forty-eight hours out of every cycle.) Thus, by having intercourse one to two days *prior* to ovulation you can ensure a good supply of sperm will be in your fallopian tube, ready for fertilization the moment your egg arrives. This not only helps increase your likelihood for getting pregnant, but improves your chances for a healthy conception.

WHEN TO MAKE LOVE: HOW TO TELL

Over the many years that I have been helping couples conceive and deliver babies, I have found that for most women ovulation routinely occurs each month, usually thirteen to fifteen days after the start of the menstrual cycle. However, this rule does not hold true for *every* patient, so I advise every woman trying to get pregnant to establish her own *personal ovulation pattern.* Utilizing one or more of several ovulation prediction methods, you can find exactly when in your cycle your eggs are being released and then use that information to calculate when you should make love.

To determine your personal ovulation pattern, use one or more of the techniques that follow.

METHOD 1: HOW YOUR BODY TEMPERATURE CAN HELP YOU GET PREGNANT

Most of my patients have found the easiest and most inexpensive way to predict ovulation naturally is to use the Basal Body Temperature (BBT) guide. Based on the principle that your body temperature rises and falls in distinct patterns connected to the fluctuations of reproductive hormones, the BBT involves taking your temperature every day for at least two months, starting on the first day of a new menstrual cycle. To establish your *fertility curve,* the time of the month when ovulation is most likely to occur, look for specific drops in body temperature, followed by elevations that remain until your next menstrual cycle.

To Get Pregnant Fast

Make love between the time your temperature drops and before it rises—a period of about twelve to twenty-four hours that usually occurs about thirteen to fifteen days after the start of your menstrual cycle.

To ensure the success of your BBT, keep a temperature chart for at least two months before attempting to establish your fertility curve, and be certain to take your temperature as soon as you wake up each morning, before getting out of bed, and before eating, drinking, or smoking. Keep a *written* record of your temperature changes; it will make your ovulation pattern clear. (Two sample charting grids are shown on page 197— one filled out as an example, the other blank for your possible use.)

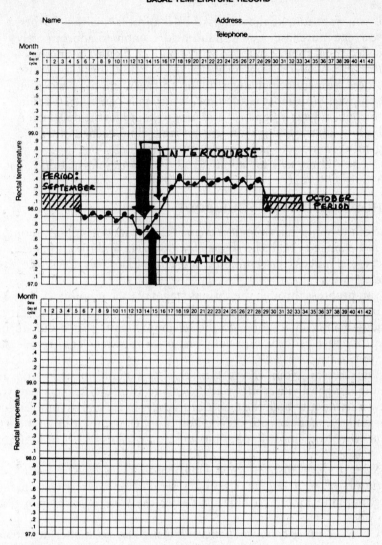

BASAL TEMPERATURE RECORD

The BBT or Basal Body Temperature Guide

Fluctuations in your basal body temperature (the temperature of your body upon waking) correlate with hormonal changes that generally indicate your most fertile time.

To get pregnant fast: always make love within the twelve- to twenty-four-hour period between the time your temperature drops (indicating ovulation is about to occur) and when it rises (indicating ovulation has occurred)—usually about twelve to fourteen days into your menstrual cycle.

By taking your BBT upon waking every morning (before you eat, drink, smoke, or get out of bed) and then recording your findings for two to three months' time, you can learn to chart your fertility curve, discovering when your most fertile time will occur in future cycles.

The High-Tech Rabbit

If you want to take the standard BBT formula one step further, you can purchase a new hand-held computer appropriately called the Rabbit. Equipped with a built-in digital thermometer that gives you readings in just sixty seconds, the Rabbit also stores temperature changes for up to twelve months and then computes your most fertile time. It also tells you when it's time to confirm your pregnancy and how to compute the due date. A built-in alarm wakes you at the same time each day with a gentle reminder to take your temperature.

The Rabbit sells for about $160. For more information call 1-800-999-1220.

METHOD 2: LISTEN TO YOUR BODY

One of the major physiological events that occurs during your monthly cycle is a change in both the shape of your cervix and the consistency of your cervical mucus, the semiliquid substance that flows down into your vagina.

As you progress through the various stages of each monthly cycle, both the quantity and quality of your mucus, and the shape of your cervix changes—mainly in response to the hormonal shifts that occur during the reproductive process, especially just prior to when eggs are released from your ovary.

For this reason, your cervix can serve as a guide to when you are ovulating. By gently inserting your finger into your vagina every day, you can learn to identify both the tactile differences in the feel of your cervical mucus and the shape of your cervix. You can then use these differences to tell you when your most fertile time will occur. Here's what to look for:

1. *Start of the menstrual cycle—mucus: dry.* This is the relative condition of your vagina starting several days after ovulation and continuing for up to nine days after the start of each menstrual cycle.
   Corresponding cervical changes: During and right after menstruation, your cervix will be in a low position. It will feel firm and have a pointy shape and be relatively easy to touch.
2. *Several days before ovulation—mucus: creamy wet.* Mucus flow starts to increase about nine days after the start of your menstrual cycle and has a smooth texture and creamy white appearance.
3. *Approaching ovulation—mucus: thin, slippery, stretchy, and clear.* As you approach ovulation (approximately thirteen to fifteen days into your cycle), your mucus takes on the appearance of egg white and has a slimy consistency. This allows it to transport sperm

quickly through your vaginal canal and into your fallopian tubes. *Corresponding cervical changes.* As you approach ovulation, your cervix will respond to rising estrogen levels by pulling slightly up and rotating forward. This places the opening in a better position for sperm passage. It might be slightly harder to reach; it will feel softer to the touch and be very wet. At this point cervical mucus is at its peak production.

Immediately following ovulation, your mucus production takes a sharp decline. Whatever is left becomes gluelike and extremely sticky, often resembling rubber cement. It remains at this consistency for two or three days and then becomes very dry again. Your cervix correspondingly drops back down again, responding to a dip in estrogen levels. It will once again feel hard and pointy.

To Get Pregnant Fast

Make love when mucus is thin, slippery, stretchy, and clear and when your cervix is rotated forward, soft and very wet to the touch.

Important ★ Important ★ Important

Do not attempt to ascertain your cervical mucus pattern while taking birth control pills or for several weeks after you discontinue their use. The hormonal fluctuations associated both with pill use and with stoppage can cause wild variations in the quality and quantity of your cervical mucus. Wait at least two months after discontinuing pill use before attempting to establish a mucus ovulation pattern.

Also important: Showering, bathing, and swimming can all temporarily alter the quality and quantity of your mucus, so be sure to make your checks prior to these activities, or wait several hours after them.

METHOD 3: HOW YOUR SALIVA CAN HELP YOU GET PREGNANT—THE NEWEST AND MAYBE THE MOST RELIABLE WAY TO PREDICT OVULATION!

The very newest method for predicting ovulation utilizes biochemical changes in your saliva. When properly analyzed, those changes can predict when your egg will be released up to *seven full days* before it is.

The device developed to do just that is called the Cue Ovulation Predictor. It works by registering electrolyte levels in your saliva (primarily sodium, calcium, and potassium), which rise and fall in particular patterns in tune with various reproductive functions. As a backup confirmation of ovulation, the Cue also electronically measures estrogen-related changes in cervical mucus. Used together, these two types of readings greatly increase the reliability of ovulation prediction.

How the Cue Works

The Cue is simple to use and requires only ten seconds of monitoring twice a day, once in the morning, once at night:

- ◆ A.M. A small spoon-shaped sensor is placed under your tongue for ten seconds. A wire connects the sensor to a small box (about the size of a cassette player), inside which a tiny computer records the electrolyte reading.
- ◆ P.M. A small tampon-shaped sensor, also connected by a wire to the computer, is placed inside your vagina for ten seconds, and the cervical mucus reading is registered.

Unlike the BBT, neither the A.M. or P.M. Cue reading requires that you limit movement prior to testing. For the A.M. reading, however, you cannot eat or drink or smoke cigarettes prior to placing the sensor in your mouth. Both A.M. and P.M. readings must be taken at the same time every day, starting at the beginning of your menstrual cycle and continuing a few days past ovulation.

The cost of the Cue is generally quite high, but the unit can be rented from the manufacturer for a reasonable fee. As another option, you can purchase a factory-sealed set of sensors for about $80, and then rent the computerized registering box.

For more information on the Cue, contact The Zetek Corporation, 794 Ventura Street, Aurora, CO 80011 (1-800-367-2837).

METHOD 4: OVULATION PREDICTOR KITS

The discovery of some key hormones involved in the ovulation process—namely FSH and LH, opened a new world of biochemical technology which made tracking egg release markedly faster, easier, and more accurate. Thus, the concept of ovulation predictor kits was born. Utilizing a series of early-morning urine samples, the ovulation predictor kits measure levels of LH, the hormone released into your system in great abundance just prior to ovulation. Adding your urine to a plastic vial filled with a chemical solution, you can watch for color changes that indicate the degree of LH being excreted from your body. The color (usually blue) ranges from light, meaning very little LH is present, to very dark, meaning your LH levels are peaking and ovulation is about to occur.

To Get Pregnant Fast

Make love within twelve to twenty-four hours after your urine solution turns its darkest color, indicating a surge in LH.

A Warning About Ovulation Predictor Kits

If you are over forty and using a commercial ovulation predictor kit, be aware that the onset of menopause can also cause elevated levels of LH, and they *do not* signify ovulation. Although most women do not experience hormonal changes indicative of menopause until they approach their late forties, it is possible to get this type of high LH level at an earlier age. For this reason, check with your doctor if your tests show elevated LH levels for longer than a day or two in midcycle.

★ Important ★ Important ★ Important

Some fertility drugs used to promote ovulation, such as Danocrine or Pergonal, can affect the results of some ovulation predictor kits. If you are on any fertility drugs, check with your doctor before purchasing a kit.

One fertility drug that usually does not affect test results is Clomid.

SEX AND CONCEPTION: HOW TO MAKE LOVE TO GET PREGNANT

In addition to having intercourse at the right time of the month (your most fertile time) how you make love can also influence both the speed of your conception—and in some cases, your ability to get pregnant at all.

In fact, the positions both you and your partner assume during and right after your lovemaking can have an enormous influence on fertility, significantly affecting the passage of sperm from your vagina to your fallopian tube.

THE SEXUAL POSITIONS THAT ENCOURAGE CONCEPTION

Because individual anatomies and certain personal biological details are different for every couple, the positions of love most effective for fertility can vary from couple to couple. Generally, however, the following guidelines have proved to be helpful to many of my patients, most of whom found that changing their sexual positions made a difference in the speed with which they could conceive.

What can make a difference? Any position that increases the natural backward tilt of your vagina can also increase your chances for conception by allowing sperm to get a good head start in the right direction. These include:

- *Male dominant, or missionary style.* This can be especially effective if a pillow is placed under your pelvic region, causing your vagina to tilt backwards.
- *Knee to chest, or rear-entry style.* This can help your partner deposit his sperm closer to your cervix and can be very effective for increasing the power of a marginal or low sperm count.
- *Lying on your side.* Many of my patients report that this can be an especially important position if either partner suffers from back problems or if the man is very overweight. By taking excess pressure off the delicate nerve endings that collect at the base of your spine, you may be able to relax more during intercourse, and that can help facilitate a speedy passage of sperm to your vagina.

HOW *NOT* TO MAKE LOVE

What are the worst sexual positions for conception?

- Sitting
- Standing
- Female dominant (woman on top)
- Bending over

These positions discourage the rapid transport of sperm and can make conception more difficult.

MORNING LOVE AND YOUR FERTILITY

Although there are no statistics to show that making love during any particular time of day will increase conception odds, sperm count is usually highest in the morning if you have not made love the night before. Morning is also the time when male hormones are at their peak, which is why many men have their strongest sexual urges in the morning upon awakening. If sperm count is a deciding factor in your fertility, then morning love *could* make the difference!

SEX AND YOUR BABY'S SEX

In addition to affecting fertilization, some research suggests that how you make love can also influence the sex of the child you create. This is said to be due to differences in the genes carried by sperm.

Sperm is divided into two types, those that carry genes for a female child and those that carry genes for a male child.

MALE SPERM ARE SAID TO BE

- Fast moving
- Good swimmers
- Small
- Easily affected by acidic vaginal secretions
- Short lived

FEMALE SPERM ARE SAID TO BE

- Slow moving
- Large and hardy
- Able to withstand acidic environments
- Able to survive longer in the female body

According to the sex selection theory, certain sexual positions, along with the depth of penetration and when in relation to ovulation you make love, can be used to encourage fertilization with either male or female sperm. While there is no guarantee that sex selection will work, many of my patients have used the following techniques to plan their families with incredible accuracy.

If you want a baby girl:

- Shallow penetration in the missionary position (man on top) will allow your partner to deposit sperm at the mouth of your cervix. This is said to favor the slower-moving female sperm.
- Avoid orgasm. This will help keep your vaginal environment highly acidic, which helps kill off the male sperm before they reach your fallopian tube. To increase the acidity of your vagina even more, use a vinegar and water douche (two tablespoons of vinegar in one quart of water) directly preceding intercourse.
- Abstain from sex on the third and fourth day prior to ovulation and begin making love two days prior to ovulation. If you are using an ovulation predictor kit, make love when the solution is darkest.

If you want a baby boy:

◆ Use deep penetration, and the rear-entry position, which will allow your partner to deposit sperm above the neck of your cervix, for fast entry into your uterus. Here the environment is more alkaline, making it easier for male sperm to survive.

◆ Douche with two tablespoons of baking soda in one quart of water just prior to making love. This will encourage an alkaline vaginal environment, enhancing the survival rate of sperm, making them stronger and able to swim faster, thus increasing the chance for conception with male sperm.

◆ Try to achieve orgasm at the same time that your partner is ejaculating. This will also help create a more alkaline vaginal environment.

◆ Your partner should avoid masturbation for four to five days, and you should both avoid intercourse until your day of ovulation. This will help ensure the highest possible sperm count and, together with the other factors, give the advantage to the fast-swimming male sperm. If you are using an ovulation predictor kit, make love twenty-four hours *after* the solution turns its darkest color.

In addition, the closer to the exact time of ovulation you make love, the better your chances of having the faster male sperm reach your egg first. If you have sex one or two days *prior* to ovulation, there is likely to be a greater abundance of hardier female sperm waiting in your fallopian tube.

HOW THE SUN CAN HELP YOU GET PREGNANT

One of the factors affecting conception that I personally find most fascinating is the role the sun has been found to play in helping you get pregnant. In one of the several new studies on the effects of the environment on fertility it was found that biological functions, including reproduction, are affected by the number of hours you spend exposed to light. Most profound in terms of your fertility is the effect of light on the regularity of your menstrual cycle. The connection, it seems, is soltriol, a steroid hormone that is commonly known as vitamin D. (Recent research has shown that it isn't a true vitamin.) According to the Department of Cell Biology and Anatomy and the Department of Pharmacology at the University of North Carolina at Chapel Hill, soltriol (also called the *hormone of light*) is manufactured in the body in response to stimulation by exposure to light and has the ability to regulate reproduction by directly interacting with receptors in the hypothalamus and pituitary glands, the uterus, oviducts, and the mammary glands, as well as in the baby's placenta and the fetal membranes.

Based on these studies, many researchers believe that, by helping your body manufacture and maintain adequate levels of soltriol, spending time in the sun *can* increase your fertility. I have recommended the sunlight method to patients with unexplained infertility, so long as they were not extremely light sensitive, and found that it can make a difference. Several who had not been able to conceive did so after taking vacations in warm, sunny climates, while several others tremendously improved the timing and the regularity of their menstrual cycles after managing to catch just a few extra hours of sunlight every week.

Conversely, I have also seen patients develop temporary infertility when their jobs deprived them of their usual amount of sunlight.

CAN YOU TRY TOO HARD TO GET PREGNANT?

Nearly every couple who comes to me for fertility counseling knows at least one other couple who, after years of unsuccessfully trying to have a baby, finally conceived—but only after they had abandoned hope. Thus the notion of trying too hard.

Is it real? Yes, it is. But only when trying turns a natural, loving desire to have a baby into a mandate filled with fear and worry and anxiety.

CAN SWEAT MAKE YOU MORE FERTILE?

One of the most interesting new theories on fertility holds that the way we smell may have an ability to encourage conception.

Although it has long been known that the scent an animal gives off when fertile attracts a mate, several new human studies have shown that the scent a man's body gives off when *he's* turned on can not only turn *you* on, but actually increase your fertility by helping you have more regular menstrual cycles.

In addition, a recent report presented to the American Chemical Society by the Monsell Chemical Senses Center in Philadelphia suggests a link between underarm chemicals and the length and timing of the menstrual cycle. Long believed to be a means of communicating sexual and social messages, underarm (and other body) odors may prove to have an important link to fertility. Researchers at the Monsell Center are examining whether these odors can influence the secretion pattern of pituitary hormones, which may in turn affect the menstrual cycle. Although it is certainly too early to draw conclusions, avoiding deodorant and perfumes prior to attempting conception may very well turn out to influence how fast you get pregnant.

GETTING PREGNANT AFTER THIRTY-FIVE

One of the questions I am most often asked is how long a couple can safely postpone childbearing without harming their chance to conceive. The answer is easy: longer than ever before! While it was once believed that any pregnancy after age thirty was unsafe and unhealthy for both mother and child, today advances in both prepregnancy and prenatal care, as well as those made in reproductive technologies, are helping couples have healthier babies, no matter when in their childbearing years they decide to conceive. In fact, as long as your body is healthy enough to withstand labor and delivery, there are laboratory techniques that can allow you to have a child at almost any age—in some cases, even after menopause! (You'll learn more about these exciting new discoveries in Chapter Twenty-One.)

However, in terms of having an *all-natural* pregnancy after age thirty-five (and by that I mean one that does not require any laboratory assistance to help you conceive) the answer to the question of extended fertility is a bit more complex.

As you have read in Part One, many factors affect your reproductive health and determine your fertility status. Moreover, because every woman's body is physiologically unique, to what age you will be able to have a natural conception depends on your personal biology. I have had patients who stopped making eggs and began menopause as early as thirty-five or forty, while others showed no signs until age forty-five or beyond.

However, because your fertile years are somewhat hereditary, you can get a good idea of your childbearing potential by checking with your mother, grandmother, or other close female relatives regarding the age at which they began to experience menopause. Your own body will also give you some early signs—missed periods, irregular cycles, hot flashes, fatigue, and mood swings. When these warning signs do begin to appear, your opportunity to conceive a child naturally is coming to a close—and even your ability to do so with laboratory assistance can be somewhat compromised. You can still get pregnant, but it's a good idea not to wait too much longer.

Over Thirty-Five: How to Have a Fast, Natural Conception

As long as you are still making eggs and you have no structural damage in your reproductive system, there is a chance you can conceive naturally. However, as you age, your eggs age too (remember, your complete supply is with you from birth). And because studies show old eggs don't generally fertilize as quickly or as easily as young eggs, very often pregnancy doesn't occur as quickly or as easily as it does when you are younger. In addition, when you are over thirty-five your reproductive hormones and organs work less efficiently, too, which can place some additional restrictions on how quickly or easily a fertilized egg will be transported, implanted, and start to grow. For all these reasons, all conception statistics (even those using laboratory assistance) drop sharply after age forty, so don't be disappointed if you don't conceive immediately after you begin trying.

The good news is that if you are over thirty-five there are steps you can take to *help you* achieve a faster, healthier, natural conception:

- ◆ Go for a preliminary fertility exam before you even try to conceive. Make sure you are free of any obvious problems like fibroid tumors, endometriosis, or blocked or damaged tubes or ovaries as a result of disease or scar tissue.
- ◆ Be checked for STDs and other diseases that can block a pregnancy, especially chlamydia and yeast infections.
- ◆ Have your partner's sperm count checked as soon as you decide to get pregnant. While a man makes new sperm every day of his life, a variety of age-related factors can take their toll on the quality and quantity of sperm he is producing and releasing.
- ◆ Pay very strict attention to all the nutritional and dietary guidelines described in Chapter Eleven. This information is important for women of all ages, but it is particularly crucial to women over thirty-five. I have seen many older patients get pregnant naturally by simply changing their eating habits, reaching their fertility weight goals, and taking vitamins.
- ◆ If you don't get pregnant after four to six months of regular unprotected intercourse (three times weekly), see a fertility specialist immediately. Although natural conception can take longer after age thirty, I do not advise that you wait. If it turns out that you need laboratory assistance to get pregnant, the younger you are (even in terms of months), the better your chances.
- ◆ Finally, make certain you choose a top-quality fertility specialist who has experience treating women over thirty-five. Even today, many reproductive specialists still routinely discourage older women from getting pregnant, so make certain you take the advice of one who regularly treats women over thirty-five.

ONE DOZEN SUPER NEW AND TIME-TESTED WAYS TO ENCOURAGE A NATURAL CONCEPTION AT ANY AGE!

Although timing love-making to coincide with ovulation is the best way to ensure conception, it isn't the only way! You and your partner can take a number of steps to encourage not only a quick pregnancy, but a healthy one. Here are twelve new, but also time-tested, ways to do just that!

1. MAKE LOVE WITH THE LIGHTS ON

In addition to the role that sunlight can play in encouraging conception, other studies have shown that artificial light, like a lamp, kept on at night can have an effect on your fertility, encouraging regular menstrual cycles and keeping ovulation on schedule. In one study a woman was able to control the regularity of her menstrual cycle for three months by simply sleeping with the light on, on the fourteenth, sixteenth, and seventeenth nights. In addition, she could increase the length of her cycle according to the number of hours the light was turned off (half a night, as opposed to a whole night).

As a result of studies like these, some researchers believe that sleeping with the lights on for several weeks, and making love in that environment as well, could encourage conception by helping to keep ovulation regulated.

2. MAKE LOVE BETWEEN OCTOBER AND MARCH

According to brand-new reports in the *British Medical Journal,* making love from October to March can *double* your chances of getting pregnant! Researchers speculate that egg quality, as well as positive changes in the uterus, can increase in direct relation to the changes in temperature, climate, and light that occur during these months.

The worst times to attempt conception? August and September. According to recent research published in the *American Journal of Obstetrics and Gynecology,* births drop dramatically during April and May, indicating that August and September may not be fruitful months in which to conceive.

3. MAKE LOVE ON YOUR BIRTHDAY

As reported in *Gynaekologe,* a respected Japanese medical journal, the fertility of some women may be season-sensitive, increasing around the time of their birthday. According to the study, making love close to the day you were born may make conception faster and easier.

4. BE TURNED ON WHEN YOU MAKE LOVE

Because being sexually stimulated can influence the flow of reproductive hormones, research indicates that couples who are very turned on when they try to conceive may have a faster, easier time getting pregnant. In addition, the very latest studies show that the sperm count of men who ejaculate when they are turned on and making love is higher and more potent than that of men who masturbate.

And, don't forget the power that simple touching and caressing can have to boost your fertility! Studies show that just twenty to forty minutes of stimulating sexual caresses prior to intercourse can increase hormone levels and encourage fertility.

In short, whatever turns both of you on is a great conception booster.

5. DON'T MAKE LOVE UNDER AN ELECTRIC BLANKET

The very latest studies show that the low voltage emitted by electric blankets may adversely affect fertility. There is also evidence that conception which takes place under an electric blanket may yield a higher rate of birth defects and miscarriage. So, if you're trying to get pregnant, let your love keep you warm!

6. MAKE LOVE CLOSE TO THE TIME OF OVULATION AND AVOID MISCARRIAGE

In a fertility study of 965 women, all of whom kept detailed records of sexual activity, it was shown that the likelihood of miscarriage decreased when conception took place at the time of ovulation. When fertilization occurred three days *after* ovulation, when eggs are still present but already on their way to disintegration, the chance of miscarriage *tripled*.

7. LIMIT MOVEMENT AFTER INTERCOURSE

By remaining in bed for twenty to thirty minutes after intercourse, preferably on your back, with a pillow under your pelvic region, you can help encourage sperm to remain in your body and flow upward toward your fallopian tubes.

8. UTILIZE FAST WITHDRAWAL

Research suggests that by withdrawing his penis immediately after releasing the first squirt of his ejaculation, your partner can increase sperm concentration and thereby improve chances for conception.

9. RETAIN SPERM IN YOUR VAGINA

Immediately after intercourse, lightly press the labia (lips) of your vagina together with your finger, and hold for several minutes. This can help keep sperm inside your vagina and ensure that what has been deposited has the opportunity to swim toward your fallopian tube.

10. AVOID ALCOHOL AND DRUGS AT THE TIME OF CONCEPTION

Although some couples have grown accustomed to increasing sexual stimulation and enjoyment through the use of alcohol and/or drugs prior to making love, I cannot emphasize enough the importance of avoiding this practice, especially at the time of conception. Mounting evidence shows that alcohol in your bloodstream or your partner's at the time of conception can have some overwhelmingly negative effects not only on your fertility, but on your baby as well. Do not use either of these substances on or around the time you plan to conceive.

11. TAKE ROBITUSSIN COUGH MEDICINE

Robitussin, which contains the active ingredient guaifenesin and helps thin the mucus in your lungs, can also alter cervical mucus, making it thinner and better able to transport sperm. Many of my own patients who were unable to conceive have helped solve their infertility problems by using this simple method. Take one to two teaspoons a day, beginning three to four days prior to when you want to conceive.

12. LIMIT INTERCOURSE AND/OR AVOID MALE MASTURBATION

Avoiding ejaculation for two to five days prior to attempting conception will increase the sperm count and ensure that your partner retains the higher percentage of perfect sperm for your conception.

A FINAL WORD ABOUT CONCEPTION

It is my hope that the suggestions in this chapter will help you obtain a fast and easy conception, but I don't want you to worry about accomplishing them. Feel calm and confident about your ability to get pregnant; feel happy and positive about being a parent. Maintaining the right emotional state is perhaps the best way to achieve a successful conception.

Relax . . . make love . . . enjoy!

· 14 ·

PREVENTING MISCARRIAGE—NOW YOU CAN!

Some of the most exciting advances in reproductive medicine are the breakthroughs for the prevention of miscarriage. Today, there are a multitude of ways your doctor can help protect your conception and you and your partner can reduce your risk of pregnancy loss even if you have miscarried in the past. Among my own patients I have seen couples who had been plagued with the frustration of seemingly unexplained recurring miscarriages conceive and deliver healthy babies, using the simplest of these preventative new treatments.

UNDERSTANDING PREGNANCY LOSS: THE LATEST NEWS

Medically called a spontaneous abortion, for most couples a miscarriage normally happens only one time. The cause is usually an isolated chromosomal abnormality, which occurs when fertilization involves a defective egg or sperm. This blighted ovum, as it is called, is simply too weak to survive. As a result, sometime in the first twenty weeks of pregnancy it detaches from the uterus and leaves the body.

Under most circumstances, the next attempt at conception is healthy. In fact, because reproductive hormones are usually at their peak just prior to a miscarriage, I often advise my patients to try for another pregnancy as soon as one month following their loss. When they do, most find this second conception is faster and easier, not to mention healthy.

211

WHEN MISCARRIAGE HAPPENS
MORE THAN ONCE

For some prospective parents, however, pregnancy loss is not an isolated event. A growing number of couples are continually plagued with what is medically called habitual abortion. For these couples, some factor either in their personal biology or in their lifestyle continually interferes with either the quality of their conceptions or the implantation process. They are, in fact, considered infertile, unable to deliver a child.

In the past, recurring miscarriage was linked primarily to two factors:

- *Structural abnormalities.* This normally means that some kind of blockage or deviation in your uterus or a weakness in your cervix is interfering with the successful implantation and/or growth and development of a fertilized egg.
- *Chromosomal abnormalities.* Here, chronically defective genetic material in your eggs or your partner's sperm continually creates embryos that are too weak to survive.

Now, however, much has changed. Although both structural and chromosomal abnormalities still account for a good number of recurring miscarriages, we now know there are a significant number of other biological reasons for pregnancy loss, including:

- Hormone imbalance
- Endometriosis
- Stress
- Diabetes
- Infection
- Sperm allergy
- Thyroid malfunction
- Immune system deficiencies

While not all women who have these problems will inevitably miscarry, there is a significant correlation between certain biological factors and a tendency toward miscarriage.

WHAT CAN INCREASE YOUR RISK OF MISCARRIAGE?

- A history of premature labor and/or premature birth
- Age—if you are over thirty
- Endometriosis
- Difficulty in conceiving
- Your mother took DES
- A history of four or more abortions
- A history of PID or repeated bouts with STDs
- Recurring urinary tract infections

Alone, and even more so in combination with some of the high-risk lifestyle factors mentioned in Chapters Five and Six (smoking and drug and alcohol use, for example), any of these biological conditions may increase your chances for miscarriage.

MISCARRIAGE ALERT: THE NEW HIGH-RISK FACTOR

A startling new discovery made by British researchers has shown that LH (the hormone responsible for ovulation) may be an important link to miscarriage.

The study, conducted by Dr. Lesley Regan, Dr. Elisabeth Owen, and Professor Howard Jacobs, all of the Rosie Maternity Hospital and University College of Medicine, Cambridge, England, involved 193 women all planning to get pregnant. After testing it was found that those women who had an elevated serum LH level *prior* to getting pregnant (tested on the seventh day of their menstrual cycle), had a miscarriage rate of 65 percent, as compared with 12 percent for those who had a normal LH reading.

Although the results of the study (recently reported in *Lancet,* a British medical journal) are still inconclusive, they indicate that having your LH level tested prior to conceiving may alert you to the need for special precautions after you conceive, including taking special medications and being especially careful to avoid high-risk factors such as cigarettes, caffeine, alcohol, and VDT terminals.

PREVENTING PREGNANCY LOSS: WHAT YOU CAN DO

In earlier chapters I showed some of the lifestyle changes you can make to help you have a healthier conception. Many of them can help you avoid miscarriage as well. Later in this chapter you will discover several more key things that you and your partner can do to help ensure your pregnancy. Self-help, however, is by no means the whole story. There are medical treatments for the prevention of miscarriage, ways that, together with your doctor, you can take complete control of your pregnancy and increase your odds to an all-time high. The following guide presents some of the newest medical information you need. I have seen all the therapies mentioned result in successful births.

HOW MANY MISCARRIAGES SPELL TROUBLE?

Most fertility specialists now agree that having three or more consecutive pregnancy losses is a sign that a serious biological malfunction may exist. I, however, have always believed that *any* pregnancy loss is a sign that a patient needs extra attention and treatment. In order to avoid future difficulties, I urge you to seek at least a preliminary fertility evaluation if you have miscarried even once.

SEVEN SUPER BREAKTHROUGHS IN MISCARRIAGE PREVENTION!

BREAKTHROUGH 1: THE IMMUNE SYSTEM BOOSTER THAT IS SAVING BABIES

Because your developing fetus is a mixture of your tissue and your partner's, under ordinary circumstances your body would recognize this combination as foreign and begin treating it much like an invading microorganism: Your immune system would manufacture antibodies to destroy it. In order to keep this from happening, nature has provided you with an automatic protective biological response to pregnancy—blocking antibodies. They keep your body from attacking your baby. You begin to manufacture them the moment you become pregnant.

When, however, a particular kind of deficiency in your immune system exists, the blocking antibodies are not made. As a result, your body views your baby as a hostile invader, and your immune system goes to work to destroy it. The result: recurring miscarriage.

How This Treatment Can Help You

While researching the causes and effects of immune system stimulation, researchers made an astonishing discovery. When the white blood cells of your partner (or any suitable donor) are injected into your body, you begin to manufacture the blocking antibody!

According to Dr. D. Ware Branch of the University of Utah College of Medicine, one of the pioneers of this treatment, once immunized with their partner's (or a donor's) white blood cells, more than 70 percent of the women studied were able to successfully conceive and deliver. Injections normally begin just prior to conception and continue for several weeks into your pregnancy.

Although widely used in Europe and currently a mainstay in fertility clinics throughout England, where researchers have found it both safe and effective, this treatment is still considered experimental in the United States. (A few researchers here have suggested further testing is needed to determine if it may slightly increase the risk of birth defects and/or low-birthweight babies.)

To locate a medical center performing white blood cell immunotherapy in your area, contact the American Fertility Society or RESOLVE, a national support group for couples with fertility problems, listed in the resource section at the end of this book.

You Might Need This Treatment If:

- ◆ You have unexplained recurring miscarriages.
- ◆ Your partner's sperm tests normal.
- ◆ You have miscarried any babies conceived via laboratory assistance, such as artificial insemination or in vitro fertilization.

BREAKTHROUGH 2: HOW BABY ASPIRIN CAN SAVE YOUR PREGNANCY

Another type of immune system deficiency, one that causes a blood-clotting disorder, may also be responsible for a significant number of recurring miscarriages. According to researchers at Jefferson Medical College in Philadelphia, when certain antibodies are present in your system, you can develop blood clots in the vessels leading to your baby's placenta, the sac by which he or she receives nourishment from your body. These clots can keep vital nutrients from reaching your baby, who, as a result, may never develop sufficiently to sustain life.

How This Treatment Can Help You

Although a variety of drugs have been used in the experimental treatment of clotting disorder, research shows that when administered under the guidance of your physician, one of the most successful, in terms of preventing miscarriage, is baby aspirin. Thought to thin your blood sufficiently to keep the nutrient-blocking clots from forming, baby aspirin also helps to keep your blood flow even and consistent, which means your baby's nourishment is also more regular.

Other studies have shown that baby aspirin may also help stimulate your immune system, strengthening your ability to manufacture the blocking antibodies and thus giving your pregnancy an extra edge of protection.

The recommended dosage is one baby aspirin daily, starting about two weeks prior to when you plan to conceive and continuing into the first trimester of your pregnancy. While the use of aspirin at any time during pregnancy was once believed to be tied to some birth defects, the latest studies reported in the *New England Journal of Medicine* have shown that taking aspirin *early* in your pregnancy is safe. A recent FDA ruling requires all products containing aspirin to carry warning labels pertaining to use in pregnancy; this warning, however, refers primarily to those effects that have a *slight* chance of occurring in the third trimester of your pregnancy and/or during delivery.

You Might Need This Treatment If:

- ◆ You have unexplained recurring miscarriages.
- ◆ You test positive for autoimmune disorders, such as rheumatoid arthritis or systemic lupus erythematosus.
- ◆ Your blood test is positive for the presence of anticardiolipin antibodies, the biochemical responsible for this condition.

BREAKTHROUGH 3: THE NATURAL HORMONE SUPPLEMENT THAT CAN SAVE YOUR PREGNANCY

One of the most common causes of miscarriage is a faulty implantation. That is, although your conception was healthy and your fetus is in good shape, it fails to adequately attach to your uterus. When this occurs, your baby cannot be properly nourished. In addition, if the implantation is exceptionally weak, normal movement is sometimes enough to shake it loose, and cause you to miscarry.

Although a number of factors can cause a faulty or weak implantation, the latest research shows one of the most common is a lack of progesterone, a hormone that is manufactured after ovulation and serves to soften and condition the lining of your uterus, making implantation healthier and stronger. When progesterone is in short supply during the second half of your menstrual cycle (this is called a luteal phase defect), your uterine lining remains rigid. This can either prevent implantation from occurring or cause any that does occur to be weak.

How This Treatment Can Help You

By taking progesterone supplements prior to conceiving, you help ensure that the amount of this hormone necessary for a healthy implantation is present in your body. In addition, progesterone supplements taken after conception can prevent miscarriage by helping to keep prostaglandin levels from rising too high. When this hormone-like substance is elevated, severe uterine cramping, similar to labor pains, can occur, causing you to expel your fetus.

Although the treatment is safe for you and your baby (no negative side effects have been reported), it's important that only *natural progesterone supplements* be used in this treatment. Most synthetic forms of this hormone (like the kind found in some birth control pills) will have no beneficial effects. However, some fertility clinics have recently reported success with hydroxyprogesterone caproate, a long-lasting synthetic progesterone.

An extra bonus: Studies show that if you use natural progesterone suppositories during the early part of your pregnancy, your baby may be more intelligent than those born to mothers who do not use this supplement.

You Might Need This Treatment If:

- Blood and/or urine tests indicate low progesterone levels during the last two weeks of any menstrual cycle.
- Your body temperature does not rise after ovulation, or it fluctuates intensely. Using the BBT guide in Chapter Thirteen, you can help detect a progesterone deficiency by watching for a significant temperature increase of about one degree after ovulation. If it does not occur, progesterone may be deficient.
- Your menstrual cycles are irregular. This can also indicate a hormone imbalance strong enough to affect your pregnancy.

BREAKTHROUGH 4: STOPPING THE BACTERIA THAT STOP A PREGNANCY

In addition to causing infertility, it has recently been discovered that certain types of bacterial infections can cause miscarriage, affecting both the quality of your egg as well as your implantation. The presence of these bacteria can also create what is called a hostile environment, which can have debilitating effects on sperm. The most common bacteria linked to pregnancy loss are those usually associated with STDs, including

- Chlamydia - T-mycoplasma - Gonorrhea - Syphilis

However, other micro-organisms, some not even visible under a microscope, can cause pregnancy loss as well.

How This Treatment Can Help You

Ideally, all infections should be treated long before you get pregnant. Unfortunately, one of the most frustrating things about the infection–miscarriage connection is that some of the bacteria responsible for pregnancy loss are difficult to detect, even with sophisticated laboratory tests. Some diseases also have no symptoms, so patients may not be aware that they are infected. For this reason, many fertility specialists now find it beneficial to routinely treat every couple with unexplained recurring miscarriages with antibiotics, both prior to conception and for the first several weeks of pregnancy, when some women are more susceptible to these infections.

The medication of choice is usually natural erythromycin because it has been found safe to use both prior to conceiving and during pregnancy. In fact, so safe and effective is this drug that many fertility clinics throughout the world now routinely prescribe natural erythromycin for any woman who has miscarried even once. I have found it to be one of the most beneficial treatments in preventing miscarriage and have used it time and again to help hundreds of patients overcome habitual pregnancy loss. The recommended dosage is 333 mg taken two to three times daily, beginning seven to ten days before you plan to get pregnant and continuing for six to eight weeks into the first trimester of pregnancy. Because bacteria linked to miscarriage can reside in your partner's body as well, as an extra precaution he too must be treated, even if he tests negative for the infections in question.

You Might Need This Treatment If:

- ♦ You or your partner are at high risk for STDs.
- ♦ You have miscarried in the past and no reason for your pregnancy losses can be found.
- ♦ Your last miscarriage was followed by a fever.

BREAKTHROUGH 5: HOW TO USE A CONDOM TO PREVENT MISCARRIAGE

In much the same way that you can be allergic to strawberries or roses, you can also be allergic to your partner's sperm. As a result, your body begins making sperm antibodies the moment he ejaculates into your vagina. Aimed at destroying what your body perceives as a deadly invader, the antibodies create an environment so hostile that it becomes difficult or almost impossible for sperm to survive. In most cases, the sperm will die, and no pregnancy will occur, which is why sperm antibodies are a leading cause of infertility. However, when your antibody reaction is mild to moderate, sperm may only be defected. The sperm is still able to fertilize an egg so conception takes place. But because the sperm *is* defective, that conception is usually too weak or too frail to survive, thus setting the miscarriage process in motion.

How This Treatment Can Help You

As devastating as a sperm allergy can be, recent research has revealed that through regular, unvarying use of condoms for up to one year (or longer) you may be able to lessen your immune system response to your partner's sperm. Working on the same principle used to treat food allergies, where abstinence can decrease sensitivity, by avoiding direct contact with your partner's sperm for as little as six to twelve months, it is now believed, you can gradually decrease your sensitivity. Condom therapy is usually accompanied by specific tests designed to measure your level of sperm antibodies at three-month intervals. When antibody production falls low enough, you are free to conceive without fear of miscarriage.

You Might Need This Treatment If:

- You have unexplained miscarriages.
- You test positive for the presence of antisperm antibodies in your cervical mucus.
- Your partner's sperm tests normal.

BREAKTHROUGH 6: HOW ONE STITCH CAN SAVE YOUR BABY!

Normally, tight bands of fibrous tissue surround your cervix, helping to keep it closed until just before you are about to deliver. When, however, due to disease, too many selective abortions, a genetic abnormality, or a multiple birth, these tissue bands become weakened, you cannot hold your baby inside. When this problem occurs, sometime in your second trimester your cervix can dilate, after which cramping will begin, and a miscarriage occurs.

How This Treatment Can Help You

By placing a stitch around your cervix (called a Shirodkar suture) about fourteen weeks into your pregnancy, your doctor can help give your uterus the extra support it needs to hold your baby inside. I have personally found this treatment to be most effective for patients who are carrying twins or triplets as a result of a laboratory-aided conception, such as in vitro fertilization. Since fertility patients can be at a higher than average risk for pregnancy loss, this treatment can increase their odds by a tremendous margin.

You Might Need This Treatment If:

- ◆ You are pregnant with more than one baby.
- ◆ You have had more than four abortions.
- ◆ A connective tissue disease has weakened your fibrous bands.
- ◆ Your doctor diagnoses a weak cervix.

BREAKTHROUGH 7: THE NEW MEDICATIONS THAT PREVENT MISCARRIAGE

For any number of reasons a pregnancy can go into premature labor, a condition in which your uterus is stimulated into contractions normally experienced only when your baby is ready to be born. Because your baby is not fully prepared to sustain life, he or she will die if forced out of your womb.

Although it was once believed that any attempt by a fetus to leave the body should be regarded as a sign of an unhealthy pregnancy, today we know this is not so. More often than not, your baby *is* healthy, and as long as he or she remains inside your body, normal development will continue.

How This Treatment Can Help You

Over the past several years a variety of medications have become available for stopping these premature uterine contractions and allowing your pregnancy to continue on its normal course. Commonly known as labor inhibitors, they are technically classified as tocolytics and include drugs like ritodrine hydrochloride and terbutaline sulfate. These medications work to relax the body's smooth muscles, the kind that line your uterus, so they stop the muscular contractions of premature labor. When administered at the onset of premature labor symptoms, they can be effective in preventing miscarriage.

Because these drugs can affect both maternal blood pressure and pulse rate, they must be administered under strictest medical supervision. They are usually begun as an I.V. solution in a hospital, with your doctor present, and monitored blood pressure readings are taken every twenty minutes for several hours. If no problems occur, the medication can be continued in tablet form at home, until roughly the thirty-seventh week of pregnancy, when your baby is considered mature enough to be delivered.

You Might Need This Treatment If:

- You have miscarried more than once in your second trimester or have had one or more premature births.
- You have experienced premature labor in the past.
- You have uterine abnormalities or fibroid tumors or were exposed to DES in your mother's womb.
- You have experienced repeated urinary tract infections.
- You have a multiple pregnancy.

ENDOMETRIOSIS AND MISCARRIAGE: AN IMPORTANT CONNECTION

If you suffer from the menstrual-related disorder called endometriosis, studies show you are three times more likely to miscarry than women who don't have this disease. Risks increase because endometrial lesions can block the fallopian tube, making egg passage difficult or impossible. When a fertilized egg remains inside your tube too long, it can simply die, or it can take root in the tube itself and start to grow. This condition, ectopic pregnancy, is the leading cause of maternal death.

In addition, because endometrial lesions emit high levels of prostaglandin, the disease can sometimes cause uterine and/or fallopian tube contractions violent enough to pass your fertilized egg from your body before it has had a chance to implant.

Fortunately, treatment for endometriosis, including medication and/or laser surgery, can usually reduce the related risk of miscarriage.

SMOKING AND MISCARRIAGE

Besides the biological factors that can affect the health of your pregnancy, new research shows there are also some outside influences capable of increasing your risk of miscarriage. The use of drugs and alcohol and exposure to environmental pollution, radiation, and chemicals in your home or workplace can have a profound effect on your pregnancy. However, the single most important lifestyle factor capable of causing a miscarriage is smoking. Avoiding cigarettes while you are pregnant is one of the surest ways to decrease your risk of pregnancy loss.

HOW SMOKING CAUSES MISCARRIAGE

Currently, the rate of miscarriage is reported to be 20 percent *higher* for women who smoke. Each time you take a cigarette, all its toxic components go directly into your baby's bloodstream, weakening his or her entire system. In addition, the nicotine in your body causes a constriction of veins and arteries, decreasing the blood flow, and thus oxygen and other important nutrients, to your baby. The more you smoke, the less nourishment and the more toxins your baby gets until he or she literally starves to death.

Later in your pregnancy, smoking can lead to *abruptio placentae,* a condition whereby your baby's placenta deteriorates and pulls away from the wall of your uterus. Depending on when in your pregnancy this occurs, either a miscarriage or premature birth results. Fortunately, quitting smoking by the fourth month of your pregnancy can help eliminate the risk of this problem.

SMOKING BEFORE PREGNANCY: THE MISCARRIAGE LINK

If you smoke prior to conceiving and at the time of conception, your baby's placenta can attach too low in your womb. Called a *placenta previa,* this condition causes inadequate blood flow to your baby and contributes to miscarriage, premature birth, and fetal death.

COFFEE, CIGARETTES, AND ALCOHOL: THE MISCARRIAGE CONNECTION

Cigarettes alone are a leading cause of pregnancy loss, but when smoking is combined with the two factors with which it is normally associated, alcohol and caffeine, your risk of miscarriage soars.

- Just two alcoholic drinks a day can significantly increase your risk of pregnancy loss.
- Consume more than 150 mg of caffeine daily (about two cups of coffee or three colas) and you are more likely to experience a miscarriage than women who consume less.

If you can't quit smoking, don't combine cigarettes with alcohol or caffeine, either before or after you get pregnant.

STRESS AND PREGNANCY LOSS

Researchers now believe that undue or prolonged physical or emotional tension can significantly reduce the supply of blood to your fetus. This, in turn, can weaken your conception and lead to miscarriage. In addition, stress may play a role in the movement of your fallopian tubes, sending them into spasms significant enough to move your fertilized egg into your uterus before the endometrium (uterine lining) is thick and/or soft enough for a healthy implantation. If this occurs, any implantation that takes place can be weak and faulty, depriving your baby of nourishment. The consequence—an implantation that is not sufficiently attached to your body and can easily be torn loose and lost.

EXERCISE AND MISCARRIAGE: WHAT YOU NEED TO KNOW

The good news here is that, for most women, moderate exercise will not harm a pregnancy. In fact, unless your implantation is extremely weak, even direct injuries to your abdomen will likely do little harm. The key, however, is moderation. Never overdo workouts while you are pregnant, or even a healthy implantation can suffer.

The connection is your body temperature, which is naturally higher when you are pregnant. Extremely vigorous workouts can quickly and easily bring body heat into the danger zone. When your body overheats, your baby overheats as well. While your system allows excess heat to escape through your skin, your baby has no such opportunity and remains hotter a lot longer. When the heat is excessive enough for a long enough period of time, as in an aerobic dance class that lasts an hour or more, your baby can grow so hot that a miscarriage spontaneously occurs.

To help guard against pregnancy loss, take the following precautions:

- Stop any vigorous exercise once you become pregnant. It is especially important to perform only *moderate* to *mild* workouts in your first trimester.
- Make certain all workout programs are preapproved by your doctor, especially after you conceive.
- If you show any signs of a weak implantation, including brown staining or bleeding *in any amount,* or, if you are at high risk for miscarriage, refrain from *any* exercise during the first trimester of your pregnancy or until your doctor says it's okay to resume working out.

ORGASM AND PREGNANCY LOSS: CAN SEX CAUSE A MISCARRIAGE?

Patients who have miscarried frequently ask whether intercourse could have caused their pregnancy loss. One of my patients was so convinced that her husband's very active sex drive had somehow caused her miscarriage, that she remained cold and sexually unresponsive to him for weeks. This, as you can imagine, was not a very advantageous situation for a couple trying to conceive their first child.

The truth is, if your body is normal and healthy, especially if you are young and your conception is strong, sex will not harm your pregnancy. However, if you are at high risk for miscarriage—if you are over age thirty, have had endometriosis, or have had difficulty conceiving—or if you have any other high-risk factors mentioned earlier, then, yes, sex during the first few weeks of your pregnancy, maybe even during the first trimester, can be harmful.

What sexual activities can harm your pregnancy the most?

- Heavy penile thrusting
- Intense pelvic activity, especially rocking
- Deep penetration
- Anal sex
- Repeated pounding on your uterus
- Use of vibrators

The motions that accompany all these activities can shake loose a weak implantation or force your fallopian tube or your uterus into a spasm that expels your fertilized egg.

In addition, because sperm contain high levels of prostaglandin, the chemical that causes the painful uterine contractions of menstrual cramps and labor, continual or frequent ejaculations into your vagina

HOW WATER BEDS CAN CAUSE A MISCARRIAGE

In a study of 1,700 births by the University of Colorado Medical Center it was found that the use of water beds during pregnancy can sharply increase your risk of miscarriage. The reason? Electrical fields present in this environment have been found to disturb fetal development.

can induce dangerous tubal or uterine contractions that can expel any implanation that is even a little weak.

Finally, orgasm, with or without penetration, can have similar negative results—*if* you are at high risk.

Should you avoid sex during the start of your pregnancy? If you are at high risk for a miscarriage, yes—for at least the first eight weeks following conception. If possible, avoid sex for the first three to four months.

IS BOTTLED WATER LINKED TO MISCARRIAGE?

> In a recent study by the California state government it was learned that women who drank bottle water had a *lower* rate of miscarriage than those who drank tap water. Why? The toxins in some tap water have been found to be dangerous to a developing fetus.

THE NEW SKIN-CARE TREATMENT THAT THREATENS YOUR PREGNANCY

Derived from vitamin A and used to treat severe cases of acne, the medication Acutane is one of the most harmful drugs connected to pregnancy problems. When taken during pregnancy, it can contribute to miscarriage, as well as causing an increase in the risk of birth defects. I strongly advise you to not to use this medication unless you have completed your family.

MISCARRIAGES AND MEN: HOW HIS BODY AFFECTS YOUR PREGNANCY

Although sperm is extremely tiny (more than a million could easily fit on the head of a pin), inside each one is a full complement of every piece of genetic material used in the making of a child. When sperm quality is good, so, too, is the chromosomal material it contains. When, for any number of reasons, a sperm is not perfect, its genetic material is also defective.

If an imperfect sperm fertilizes even the most perfect egg, the conceptus can be defective. When this happens, your baby can be born with birth defects, or your pregnancy can end in miscarriage.

Since all men produce some defective sperm every day, there is no way to completely eliminate the threat of male-related miscarriages or birth defects. However, because so many outside factors and individual health concerns are capable of affecting sperm quality, there are many things a man can do to promote a higher percentage of perfect sperm, including:

- Refrain from drinking alcohol at least forty-eight to seventy-two hours prior to conception
- Increase his vitamin C intake to 1,000 mg daily and B complex to 100 mg daily for two weeks prior to conception
- Avoid tight underwear and tight pants for at least one week prior to conceiving
- Be checked for STDs, especially for T-mycoplasma
- When possible, avoid contamination with environmental toxins, especially lead, ethyl alcohol, and organic solvents
- Avoid x-rays
- Quit smoking
- Avoid drugs

By taking a few simple precautions in the weeks and months prior to when you want to conceive, your mate can help increase not only his potency, but his ability to help you deliver a perfect child.

TWENTY-ONE SUPER EASY WAYS TO DECREASE YOUR RISK OF MISCARRIAGE BEFORE AND AFTER YOU CONCEIVE

WHAT TO DO BEFORE YOU GET PREGNANT

1. Take one to two prenatal vitamins (or two high-potency multi-vitamins) daily, starting three months prior to conception.
2. Quit smoking.
3. Limit alcohol consumption: no more than three drinks per week in the month prior to getting pregnant. No alcohol forty-eight hours before conceiving.
4. Examine yourself weekly for any signs of STDs, especially any unusual vaginal discharges with an unpleasant odor. Report any suspicious signs to your doctor, and get treatment immediately.
5. Make certain your doctor checks you for the following medical conditions linked to miscarriage:

- Diabetes
- Hormone imbalance
- Chlamydia
- T-mycoplasma
- Thyroid malfunction
- Toxoplasmosis
- Rubella (German measles)

6. Have your partner checked for

  ◆ Low sperm count   ◆ Sperm quality   ◆ T-mycoplasma

7. Seek genetic counseling, especially if you have had more than three miscarriages and no cause can be found.
8. Have a hysterosalpingogram (x-ray of your uterus and tubes) to determine if blockages or other abnormalities capable of causing a miscarriage exist.

WHAT TO DO AFTER YOU ARE PREGNANT

9. Check with your doctor about taking 333 mg of erythromycin daily for six weeks to reduce the possibility of infections linked to miscarriage.
10. Continue taking prenatal vitamins.
11. Stop all alcohol consumption.
12. Avoid use of any products containing caffeine.
13. Avoid all sources of radiation, including VDTs, electric blankets, heating pads, water beds, color TV (sit at least ten feet away from the front *and* the back at all times), microwave ovens, airport or other security x-rays, and medical x-rays.
14. Sleep on your left side to increase blood flow to your baby.
15. Avoid exceptionally strenuous exercise.
16. If your doctor determines you have an incompetent cervix, you should receive a Shirodkar suture no later than your fourteenth week of pregnancy.
17. Limit medication to those items absolutely necessary, and avoid use of any recreational drugs.
18. With your doctor's permission, take one baby aspirin daily for the first eight to ten weeks of your pregnancy.
19. Avoid heavy lifting.
20. Avoid sex for six to eight weeks after conceiving.
21. Receive injections and/or use suppositories of natural progesterone for the first eight weeks of pregnancy.

YOU CAN STOP A MISCARRIAGE!

While it was once believed that any attempt by a fetus to leave a mother's body was a sign that the pregnancy was not a healthy one, this is no longer the case. Today, studies show that in many instances of impending miscarriage the baby is healthy, so all possible steps should be taken to prevent a pregnancy loss. First and most important, you must know the warning signs of miscarriage and report them to your doctor immediately:

MISCARRIAGE: THE WARNING SIGNS

- Blood spotting (more than a slight pink stain; brown stains are of special concern)
- Bleeding in any intensity
- Cramping, no matter how mild
- Dizziness
- Burning headache
- Swelling of joints
- Excessive nausea or vomiting
- Fever
- Extreme or especially sudden fatigue
- Fainting
- Severe or sudden backache
- Sudden loss of pregnancy symptoms

WHAT TO DO WHEN SYMPTOMS START

When any of the signs of miscarriage appear, you must call your doctor immediately. It is likely that he or she will ask you to come to the office or the hospital for an examination.

The first step is usually a pelvic exam to determine if your cervix is still closed. Next, a sonogram may be given to determine the exact environment of your uterus and to see if your baby is healthy. Finally, you should be given a blood test to measure your levels of human chorionic gonadotropin (hCG), the hormonal indication of pregnancy.

If your cervix is still closed, beta hCG levels are elevated, and your sonogram shows that your baby is okay, your pregnancy is said to be in a state of threatened abortion, and there is a good chance that your baby can be saved *if* you take a few simple precautions:

- Get plenty of bed rest. If possible, remain in bed for at least twenty-four to forty-eight hours.
- Elevate your feet as much as possible.
- Lie on your left side to increase blood flow to your baby.
- Stay in close touch with your doctor

Your doctor should administer an injection of natural progesterone, followed by treatment with natural progesterone suppositories, or additional injections.

Talk to your doctor about prescribing 333 mg of erythromycin twice a day for two weeks to ward off any infections.

If additional symptoms appear or if problems subside and then begin again, call your doctor immediately. If heavy bleeding persists and you can't reach your doctor, go directly to the nearest hospital emergency room and tell them you are pregnant.

IF YOU DO MISCARRY: TREATMENTS TO HELP YOU CONCEIVE AGAIN

To ensure healthy pregnancies in the future, make certain you receive the proper treatment and care after your miscarriage. Depending on the type of pregnancy loss you experience and when in your gestational term your loss occurs, your miscarriage will be classified in one of three distinct categories, each with its own treatment.

1. *The complete abortion.* When this occurs, the placenta has completely torn away from your uterine wall and your fetus is fully expelled into your vagina. Normally, bleeding will slow down and eventually stop, all pain will subside, and your uterus will begin contracting, returning to its normal shape and size. When this occurs, there is usually no residual tissue left, and your miscarriage is said to be complete. Although this determination must be made by your doctor, normally no further treatment is needed.

2. *The incomplete abortion.* Although a miscarriage has occurred, your placenta may still be partly attached to your uterus, and/or remnants of fetal tissue may be left inside. Because of this, your uterus cannot contract as it normally should, and the blood flow resulting from the miscarriage process cannot be stopped. As a result, severe bleeding, sometimes leading to shock, can occur. Also, fetal tissue that is not completely discharged can lead to infection and create blockages that can cause infertility. The best treatment is a suction evacuation followed by a D&C, which surgically scrapes your uterus and removes all remaining fetal tissue.

3. *Missed abortion.* This occurs when your fetus dies sometime before your twentieth week of pregnancy but remains inside your body. There was likely no bleeding or pain, and your cervix was not dilated and remains closed. The first signs of a missed abortion are the absence of obvious pregnancy symptoms, along with lack of weight gain, decrease in breast size, and lack of fetal movement. A pregnancy blood test (hCG) and a sonogram will help confirm a missed abortion, which always requires a suction evacuation or D&C as soon as a diagnosis is made.

WARNING: NEVER DIAGNOSE YOUR OWN MISCARRIAGE

Because it is vital that your miscarriage be accurately categorized and treated, never try to diagnose your own pregnancy loss. Seek medical attention whenever you believe your pregnancy is in jeopardy, and get the proper follow-up care after a miscarriage occurs. This not only could save your baby but it might preserve your future fertility as well.

GETTING PREGNANT AGAIN

Even if it turns out that you do lose more than one pregnancy, don't give up hope. I recently treated a patient who had miscarried twelve times but wouldn't give up. After no fewer than five doctors had told her it was hopeless, we discovered she was harboring a little-known (and hard-to-diagnose) parasite. Once the infection had been cleared (it took just fourteen days of antibiotic treatment), she conceived naturally, and delivered a full-term, healthy baby!

III

♦

IF YOU DON'T GET PREGNANT RIGHT AWAY...

How Science Can Help You Conceive!

♦

• 15 •

CAN I HAVE A BABY?

How to Tell

*B*ecause information on infertility largely focuses on the situation of older couples, many young men and women don't even realize they could have a problem.

How many times have you heard the following statements from well-meaning friends and family, maybe even from your own doctor?

- Late motherhood runs in our family. Just keep trying.
- You're too young to have fertility problems. Stop worrying and you'll get pregnant.
- You were pregnant once, you'll get pregnant again. There's nothing wrong.
- You can't rush nature. It has to take its course.

While it's true that not everyone's body works at the same speed, and some couples take longer than others to conceive, still, when nature takes its course, pregnancy should occur in less than a year. If you don't get pregnant within this time frame, it has been my experience that some factor requiring at least minor treatment probably exists.

How can you tell if you might have a problem? The best way to start is by listening to your own body.

HOW TO TEST YOUR OWN FERTILITY

Because your monthly menstrual cycle is at the core of all your reproductive functions, it can serve as one of the most effective barometers

233

of your fertility. By watching for signs of irregularity (bleeding disorders, abdominal pain, backaches, emotional swings, or faulty timing), you'll likely discover potential reproductive problems.

YOUR MENSTRUAL BAROMETER: WHAT TO LOOK FOR EVERY MONTH

Although the menstrual cycle differs at least slightly in every woman, there are guidelines you can use to tell if your reproductive system is functioning properly.

Cycle Regularity

One of the best signs that everything is okay is when your cycles occur in a regular, *cyclical* fashion. In a normal menstrual cycle

- ◆ Your period can fall anywhere between twenty-six and thirty-three days, with twenty-eight days being the average.
- ◆ Bleeding begins in approximately the same number of days every month.
- ◆ While occasional timing irregularities are normal, cycles should re-regulate within two months.

Fertility Alert. Periods that are erratic, arriving in a different number of days each month, or any prolonged or significant *change* in the length of time between periods may indicate a fertility problem. Also note if the time between cycles is extraordinarily short or long, even if it's the same every month. Lack of a menstrual cycle for more than three months can also be an important symptom of a fertility problem.

Regular Bleeding Patterns

How much you bleed and for how long, as well as the consistency of your menstrual blood, can be good indicators of uterine health and hormonal function. A normal menstrual flow should

1. Start light and can be sporadic on day one
2. Increase in intensity on day two
3. Taper down by the end of day three
4. End light by day four
5. Taper off, with light staining, on days five and six

In addition, your blood flow should be smooth and even, and free of clots.

Fertility Alert. Excessive bleeding, bleeding for longer than six days, blood flow that is heavy for more than three days, or large volumes of blood loss. Equally important is a blood flow that is scanty or ends abruptly after just one or two days. In addition, a flow that is *watery* or light in color or, conversely, one that is thick and filled with clots can also signal a need for medical attention.

MENSTRUAL PAIN AND YOUR FERTILITY

While every woman has an individual threshold of pain, you should feel only minimal discomfort when you are menstruating. If you experience undue abdominal cramping, nausea, vomiting, dizziness, backache, headaches, or any other significant physical or emotional symptom just prior to, during, or right after the onset of bleeding, see your doctor.

Since pain and its accompanying symptoms can often be among the first signs of impending reproductive difficulties, early diagnosis and treatment is essential.

OVULATION: ANOTHER IMPORTANT SIGN

Although your menstrual cycle is a very good barometer of many reproductive functions, the one thing it cannot indicate is whether you are ovulating (releasing eggs from your ovary) on a regular basis. It was once believed that as long as a woman menstruated, she ovulated, but we now know this is not so. In fact, I have seen a good number of patients who had seemingly normal, regular cycles but upon closer examination were discovered not to be releasing any eggs.

To begin checking your body for specific signs that you are regularly releasing eggs, use the ovulation prediction methods described in Chapter Thirteen, including the BBT (temperature) guide, inspection of cervical mucus, and, if necessary, an ovulation predictor kit.

Be certain to record your findings for at least three consecutive months, and if possible combine readings from two or more methods used simultaneously to obtain the most accurate information about your body. While it's sometimes possible to have even distinct physical signs of ovulation without any egg release, if two or more prediction methods indicate ovulation, then it's likely you don't have a problem in this area.

If, however, more than twelve months of unprotected intercourse does not yield a pregnancy, ovulation failure should be checked along with other causes of infertility.

HOW YOUR FAMILY HISTORY CAN PREDICT YOUR FERTILITY

In addition to the biological signs of fertility that listening to your body can provide, other important indications of your reproductive potential can come in the form of a family health history. While not all fertility-related reproductive problems are inherited (or inheritable), I have found that a significant number of factors capable of affecting conception do run in families.

If you are currently having problems getting pregnant, or even if you are just thinking about conceiving and don't know if a problem could exist, it's a good idea to become familiar with the health history of close female family members, like your mother, sisters, grandmother, aunts and cousins. I encourage all my patients to speak openly with relatives about whether they had any problems conceiving and try to discover a history of any inheritable fertility-related disorders, especially

- Endometriosis
- PMS
- Fibroid tumors
- Ovarian cysts

SOME IMPORTANT QUESTIONS TO ASK YOUR MOTHER

In addition, it's a good idea to ask your mother (and, if possible, your grandmother) specific questions about her reproductive history:

- How long did it take her to conceive her first child?
- Did she have any miscarriages, and if so, how many?
- Did she ever have an ectopic (or tubal) pregnancy?
- Were menstrual irregularities or cramps a problem?
- At what age did she begin menstruating, and, if applicable, at what age did menopause start?
- Did she ever take DES (a synthetic female hormone widely used in the 1950s to help control miscarriage and linked to reproductive problems in offspring)?

TAKE CHARGE OF YOUR FERTILITY

One of the most important steps you can take to make the most of your childbearing years is to seek the help of your doctor *as soon as you discover you might have a problem getting pregnant,* certainly if more than twelve consecutive months of regular (three times weekly) un-protected intercourse does not yield a pregnancy. Although it can take some couples longer than a year to conceive, if you do have a problem, the longer you wait, the less chance you have of conceiving naturally. I have seen a number of patients who, had they sought help sooner, could have solved their fertility problems much faster and easier. A few patients lost all chance to conceive naturally because they waited just *six months* too long before seeking help.

While you don't have to visit a fertility specialist, you should consult with your gynecologist and be rechecked for some of the factors included in your preconception exam:

- ◆ Chlamydia, T-mycoplasma, and other STDs
- ◆ Fibroid tumors
- ◆ Ovarian cysts
- ◆ Diabetes
- ◆ Thyroid malfunctions
- ◆ Endometriosis

Any or all of these conditions can develop in a relatively short amount of time.

THE FERTILITY WORKUP

In certain instances, especially when your menstrual barometer or ovulation signs are abnormal, it may be a good idea for your doctor to proceed with some elementary fertility testing, especially blood tests for the following reproductive hormones:

- ◆ *Estrogen.* This test should be performed right before ovulation, when, during the normal course of events, levels should be high. Low estrogen can mean you are not ovulating, a condition that can be treated with fertility drugs, as explained later in this book.
- ◆ *Progesterone.* An erratic BBT after ovulation and/or a history of miscarriage could indicate this hormone is low. You should be tested about eight to ten days prior to the onset of your menstrual cycle, a time when levels should be surging. Deficiencies can be easily treated with natural progesterone suppositories.
- ◆ *FSH and LH.* If you are over thirty-five and the possibility of premature menopause exists, you need these tests as well. They are performed on the first or second day following the onset of your period, when during your childbearing years, levels should be low. If you are starting premature menopause, treatment with fertility drugs can often reverse the process.

THE FERTILITY X-RAY

Depending on the results of your blood tests and pelvic exam, your doctor may want to order a hysterosalpingogram, a special x-ray of your reproductive tract, to help determine more precisely the condition of your uterus and fallopian tubes. The test begins by injecting an ultrasensitive dye through your vagina, into your cervix, and out through your uterus and fallopian tubes. Tracing the flow of the liquid, the x-ray visualizes the interior of these organs and shows any blockages or malformations. What can a hysterosalpingogram reveal?

- Tubal scar tissue resulting from endometriosis, PID, or a previous ectopic pregnancy
- Tubal adhesions formed from infection or a ruptured appendix, even one that occurred in your youth
- Submucous fibroid tumors (inside your uterus)
- Active endometrial lesions in your tubes or uterus
- Structural abnormalities like a misshapen or deviated uterus
- Uterine adhesions due to a molar pregnancy or an improperly performed cesarean section, myomectomy, diagnostic D&C, or abortion
- Polyps

When the liquid dye flushes completely through your tubes and into your abdominal cavity, your doctor knows that your fimbria (the fingerlike ends of your tubes) are free and clear, able to pluck your egg from its shell and carry it inside your tube for fertilization. If the fluid does not easily pass through your system, or if it collects in tiny pockets inside your uterus or tubes, one or more problems may exist.

If you have blockages, several new types of fast and easy fertility surgeries (discussed in the next chapter) are available to help restore your childbearing options.

SOME REALLY GOOD NEWS

About 30 percent of all women with unexplained infertility and no other abnormalities get pregnant after a hysterosalpingogram, even when no treatment is given. It is assumed the procedure itself helps to clear away minute blockages that may have kept sperm and egg from successfully meeting.

MORE WAYS TO DISCOVER YOUR FERTILITY POTENTIAL

Although for most of my patients the above-mentioned tests reveal the nature of their fertility problems, sometimes I have found it necessary to perform a more advanced workup before an accurate diagnosis can be made. Your doctor might therefore recommend one of the following procedures to rule out key reproductive problems.

THE ENDOMETRIAL BIOPSY

For this test your doctor removes a tiny piece of your endometrium (the lining of your uterus) and tests it for postovulatory development. The biopsy is performed two to four days prior to the expected onset of your menstrual bleeding. If you have ovulated, your endometrium will be at a specific stage of development at this time.

The test is relatively simple and is usually done without anesthesia, often right in your doctor's office. However, it can cause you to have mild uterine cramping both during the procedure and for several hours after, and you may also experience some spot bleeding for a few days, so it's a good idea not to schedule any activities for twenty-four to forty-eight hours afterward.

THE CERVICAL EXAM

This test was designed to help evaluate the amount and consistency of your cervical mucus, as well as the external opening of your cervix. The purpose is to confirm that your mucus is the right consistency and quality to promote fast and easy sperm travel and that your cervix provides an adequate gateway for the passage of sperm to your fallopian tubes.

The test is performed by inserting a speculum into your vagina, and then using a catheter (a thin tube) to aspirate a mucus sample for a laboratory examination.

Possible causes of cervical mucus abnormalities include low estrogen levels, cervical infection and certain medications.

THE POSTCOITAL TEST

Sometimes you may have enough cervical mucus, but what you produce is incompatible with your partner's sperm, creating a hostile environment that renders the sperm immotile (unable to move). The result: you cannot conceive. To test for this problem, your doctor will ask you to refrain from having sex for two days and then to have intercourse, without a lubricant, one to four hours before your office visit.

Using a catheter, your doctor will aspirate some of the mucus from your cervical canal to measure it for not only quality and quantity, but the quantity and quality of the sperm it contains, checking specifically if the sperm are motile.

This test should be performed in the middle of your cycle, as close to ovulation time as possible.

Important note: If this problem *is* diagnosed, further sperm antibody studies may be necessary to fully assess the problem. In addition, I have found that condom therapy (the same kind used to prevent miscarriage, described in Chapter Fourteen) can often help in overcoming this problem.

The best solution, however, is usually sperm washing and intrauterine insemination, two forms of laboratory assistance you will read more about later in this book.

THE LAPAROSCOPY

If no reasons for your fertility problems can be found, your doctor may elect to perform a laparoscopy, a light surgical procedure that provides a direct look inside your pelvic cavity. A complete report on this procedure and the results you can expect are found in Chapter Sixteen.

DON'T FORGET YOUR PARTNER!

In addition to the preliminary tests you are taking, don't forget that your partner needs to be tested *at the same time*. His preliminary workup should include at the very least a sperm count and bacterial culture, especially for STDs. In most cases, your doctor can perform these tests. In the event that he/she chooses not to, your partner should ask his internist for help.

IS IT TIME TO SEE A FERTILITY SPECIALIST? HOW TO TELL

In many instances your gynecologist may be able to perform most, if not all, of the tests for a preliminary fertility workup. In some cases he or she may also be a trained fertility expert, able to take you further down the road, with more advanced testing and treatment. If, however, your doctor does not specialize in fertility problems, you may want to consider a specialist right from the start, especially if your personal biological signs indicate a problem might exist.

In addition, if your doctor refuses to test you for fertility problems or wants to perform only the bare minimum of tests, or if your results are negative, and your doctor simply urges you to keep trying, consider seeing a specialist, or at least get a second opinion from another gynecologist, preferably not one in group practice with your doctor.

IF YOU DO DECIDE TO SEEK HELP . . .

If you and your partner decide to see a specialist, remember to bring along the results of any tests that either of you has previously taken, including all x-rays and scans. If tests have been performed within a six-month period of your visit, there is no need to repeat these often costly procedures. Any doctor who refuses to look at previous test results and *insists* on repeating *all* procedures should be viewed with a skeptical eye.

Likewise, if your fertility specialist dismisses you after a exceptionally short visit (and especially if he or she doesn't even bother to examine you), claiming that nothing can be done to help you, don't get discouraged. *Look for another doctor.*

I can't tell you the number of patients I have successfully treated after not one, but two, three, or even four doctors had told them there was no hope.

The point to remember is this: Don't give up on your childbearing rights without first learning *all* your fertility options. Don't take "no" for an answer from your gynecologist, your fertility specialist, or even your mate! Remember, too, if a problem *is* discovered, a plethora of new fast and easy treatments are available to help you overcome it. In addition, a wide variety of new medications can help encourage your fertility and increase your childbearing options. So don't be afraid to question your fertility—and don't waste time wondering about it! Take charge and get the answers you deserve!

· 16 ·

THE NEW FERTILITY SURGERIES

Natural Conception Made Fast and Easy

Where it once required costly hospital stays and traumatic incisions to treat even the simplest fertility problems, now, thanks to new surgical techniques and instruments, laser technology, new light anesthesia, and new postoperative medications, some of the most seemingly complex fertility problems can be solved quickly and easily, often right in your doctor's office. Many fertility-restoring procedures are so simple that you can be back to your normal routine in just twenty-four hours. In many instances you can conceive naturally just weeks later.

CAN FERTILITY SURGERY HELP YOU?

Although new medications are making some fertility procedures unnecessary, I have found that for many of my patients, surgery is still the fastest, easiest route to a natural conception. It can help if your doctor diagnoses one or more of the following conditions:

- *Cervical and vaginal abnormalities.* These include structural problems within your cervix and/or vagina, including congenital malformations and obstructions such as cysts, tumors, adhesions, or scar tissue, which can keep sperm from reaching your fallopian tube.
- *Uterine abnormalities.* This category covers congenital malformation affecting the shape or size of your uterus, including uterine septum,

in which an excess wall of tissue divides this organ into two parts. Also included are submucous fibroid tumors (which grow inside your uterus) and scar tissue or adhesions resulting from endometriosis or PID. These problems normally cause infertility by interfering with a healthy implantation and/or the subsequent growth and development of your baby. Problems in the uterus can also increase your risk of miscarriage.

◆ *Fallopian tube abnormalities.* These include blockages inside the tube (resulting from infection, ectopic pregnancies, or endometriosis), as well as damaged fimbria (tubal ends), internal tubal scar tissue, and adhesions. Among the most common causes of infertility, tubal problems could keep sperm from reaching your egg, or an egg that has been fertilized may not be able to reach your uterus.

◆ *Ovarian abnormalities.* The most common problem here is cyst formation, especially that caused by endometriosis. This can interfere with egg production and ovulation.

DO YOU NEED FERTILITY SURGERY? HOW TO TELL

If your fertility blood tests and your pelvic exam do not provide a reason why you can't get pregnant, the possibility of a structural problem should be investigated. The quickest, easiest method is an endoscopy. In this diagnostic technique, various telescope-like devices are used to view your internal organs. Three basic endoscopic procedures are used in conjunction with fertility problems:

◆ Culdoscopy   ◆ Hysteroscopy   ◆ Laparoscopy

I use all three in my fertility practice and have found great success with each of them.

A TIME-SAVING, MONEY-SAVING WAY TO SAVE YOUR FERTILITY

Perhaps the most important benefit of endoscopy is that it often allows your doctor to immediately treat some problems as they are being diagnosed.

This can save you not only the trauma of a second incision, but also the expense and the recovery time of multiple procedures—which is something my patients always have appreciated.

In many instances x-rays, and recently videos, can be taken through endoscopic instruments, providing a record of everything your doctor sees. This can also save time and money if you seek a second opinion or if you need to change doctors. Be sure to ask the physician whether your tests are being recorded. If they are, they should be a permanent part of your medical records, accessible to you.

To help you understand a little more about how these new procedures can help you get pregnant, I have prepared the following short guide.

CULDOSCOPY

This procedure is used primarily to study the condition of your uterus, fallopian tubes, and ovaries. It can help determine any abnormalities in shape or size and detect early signs of ovarian disease, including cysts and tumors.

Although its surgical applications are limited, I have successfully used culdoscopy to remove small amounts of scar tissue and adhesions and to perform ovarian biopsies.

How It's Done

First, you are sedated and then positioned on a procedure table. Your head is placed sideways on a pillow, and your arms are folded under your chest. Your knees are drawn up so that you are in a semi-kneeling position. This helps place your vagina in a backward position, making the exam easier and more accurate.

Once the position has been assumed, your doctor places a speculum inside your vagina to hold it open and makes a small internal incision just above your cervix. Here, he/she inserts an instrument called a culdoscope, a type of telescopic device that allows a study of the back surface of your uterus, fallopian tubes, and ovaries.

By inserting several types of instruments next to the culdoscope, your doctor can also perform several surgical procedures.

Precautions

A culdoscopy should never be performed when you have any of the following conditions:

- ◆ Peritonitis
- ◆ PID
- ◆ Intestinal obstructions
- ◆ Unstable cardiovascular system
- ◆ Severe endometriosis

Complications can include infection and bleeding from the puncture site.

HYSTEROSCOPY

This procedure is used to help detect abnormalities in the shape or structure of your uterus and to identify the presence of scar tissue or adhesions, especially those caused by past abortions, IUD use, uterine infections, or a D&C (a surgical scraping of the uterus). In most cases the scar tissue can also be removed during the hysteroscopy. In addition, this procedure can help diagnose and sometimes repair a uterine septum.

Hysteroscopy has also been used to determine the cause of abnormal bleeding and to detect the presence of fibroid tumors. Those smaller than three millimeters can also be removed during this same procedure.

Finally, a hysteroscopy is used to evaluate the condition of your fallopian tubes and to help determine the existence of an ectopic pregnancy.

How It's Done

After placing you under a light anesthetic or sedative, your doctor inserts a thin fiberoptic telescoping rod into your vagina, through your cervical canal, and up into your uterus. Your doctor then distends your uterus by injecting a gas, such as carbon dioxide, or a liquid solution that helps push the walls of the organ apart, allowing a better view. Inserting additional instruments, your doctor can perform the surgical procedures mentioned above.

Precautions

When performed for fertility purposes, this procedure is best done about two weeks after the start of your menstrual cycle. One of the most significant advances made in hysteroscopy has been the development of ultrafine instruments, making the procedure cleaner, simpler, and faster, and decreasing the need for heavy anesthesia. Still, a hysteroscopy should not be done during your menstrual period or if any of the following conditions exist:

- A reproductive infection
- Profuse uterine bleeding
- Pregnancy
- A recent uterine perforation
- Known cervical cancer

LAPAROSCOPY

The most common and beneficial of all endoscopic procedures, a laparoscopy allows a direct view of all your pelvic organs, including your uterus, fallopian tubes, and ovaries, as well as an opportunity to perform a number of important surgical procedures. It is most often used for

- Evaluation of ovarian disease, possible genital abnormalities, and tubal competence
- Differentiating between a fibroid tumor and a cyst
- Classification and removal of endometriosis
- A second look at previous fertility surgery
- Evaluation of a uterine perforation that may have resulted from an abortion
- Biopsies of tubes, ovary, and uterus
- Removal of adhesions
- Aspiration of ovarian cysts
- Removal of an ectopic pregnancy

It is also used for the egg retrieval process necessary for in vitro fertilization and the GIFT procedure, and for positioning the egg and sperm during the actual GIFT procedure (see Chapters Twenty and Twenty-One).

How It's Done

After sedating you with a mild, general anesthesia, your doctor makes a small incision inside your navel (it leaves no scar).

FERTILITY SURGERY:
IT DOESN'T HAVE
TO MEAN
HOSPITALIZATION

In the not so distant past, even the most minor procedures routinely required at least a one-night stay in the hospital. Today, many fertility operations can be safely performed on an outpatient basis:

- Laparoscopy
- Diagnostic D&C
- Hysteroscopy
- Coldoscopy
- Endometrial biopsies
- Cervical and vaginal biopsies
- Minor vaginal surgery

Your abdomen is then inflated with a small amount of carbon dioxide and you are positioned with your head slightly lower than your pelvis. This will help your bowels fall away from your pelvic organs, allowing a clearer view.

Into the small incision your doctor inserts the laparoscope, a long, thin, telescoping wand through which he or she can view your organs. Sometimes a probe is also inserted; this is a medical instrument used to manipulate your organs for a better view.

If the situation warrants, your doctor will make a small second incision in your lower abdomen, directly above your pubic bone, leaving no visible scar. With the use of other surgical instruments, such as the recently introduced laser knife, your doctor can perform surgery and obtain biopsies.

With one of the new fiberoptic light sources, tiny cameras attached to the laparoscopy instruments can photograph and even videotape the entire procedure.

TUBAL SURGERY: MORE WAYS TO HELP YOU GET PREGNANT FAST

While a great many fertility problems can be simply and easily remedied via endoscopic procedures, sometimes a slightly more complex kind of surgery is needed, especially when extensive tubal damage has been diagnosed.

Although a few short years ago problems involving the fallopian tube were considered irreversible, today this is no longer the case. Thanks to the advent of microsurgery (in which delicate operations are performed while the surgeon peers through a microscope) and laser surgery (a totally bloodless form of operating), a vast array of tubal surgeries are being safely and easily performed. If your doctor diagnoses fallopian tube damage, one of the following tubal surgeries can probably help you.

SALPINGOSTOMY

This operation is most often performed to remove *significant* blockages in your fallopian tubes, including those caused by *extensive* adhesions and/or scar tissue (on the inside or the outside) that can develop due to multiple incidence of PID or severe endometriosis. Depending on the degree of damage, the success rate for conception after this procedure varies, but the average is about 26 percent.

FIMBRIOPLASTY

This procedure corrects damage to your fimbria, (the finger-like ends of your fallopian tube) usually caused by infection. Mild to moderate damage can be successfully repaired, but acute damage should be left alone; conception in such a case should be achieved via a laboratory procedure like in vitro fertilization or the GIFT procedure (see Chapters Twenty and Twenty-One).

ANASTOMOSIS

This is used to reverse a voluntary tubal sterilization. It is also sometimes done to repair congenital malformations, to remove remnants of an ectopic pregnancy, or to remove a cyst or tumor from inside your tube.

Depending on your problem, when skillfully performed this surgery can increase your chances of getting pregnant by up to 50 percent and decrease your risk of ectopic pregnancy by almost 80 percent. The success rates vary according to the portion of your tube that requires surgery and the size of the section affected.

TUBAL REIMPLANTATION

This corrects a condition in which the portion of your fallopian tube closest to your uterus is blocked and cannot be opened surgically. It involves detaching the tube from your uterus, removing the damaged section, and then reattaching it.

THE BRAND-NEW PROCEDURE THAT SAVES FALLOPIAN TUBES

In addition to the standard surgical procedures, there is now a brand-new way to help treat blockages in your fallopian tube.

Utilizing the same medical technology used to clear clogged arteries that lead to your heart, it is called *transcervical balloon tuboplasty*.

HOW A BALLOON CAN SAVE YOUR FERTILITY

Developed in Chicago by Dr. Edmund Confino, a transcervical balloon tuboplasty utilizes a long, thin plastic catheter into which a thin guide wire has been placed. At the tip of the catheter is a balloon. The entire structure is inserted into your abdomen via a tiny incision and is then carefully guided into your fallopian tube.

Once the wire reaches the obstruction, your doctor inflates the balloon, which in turn pushes against the sides of the tube, causing it to expand and thus opening the blockage. The balloon is inflated again and the procedure repeated as many times as necessary to clear the length of the tube.

Although there are no formal statistics on how long the tube remains unblocked or the rate of pregnancy after this procedure, results look promising.

THE FERTILITY SURGERY THAT IS REPLACING HYSTERECTOMIES

As you read earlier in this book, fibroid tumors can be a major source of fertility problems, decreasing your chances for a healthy implantation and increasing your risk of miscarriage by a significant margin. In the not so distant past (and in many instances still today), the treatment for fibroid tumors meant the end of a woman's reproductive potential. Believing that a hysterectomy (the surgical procedure that removes *all* the reproductive organs) was the only way to manage these troublesome but rarely dangerous growths, many doctors routinely destroyed a woman's fertility just to remove a fibroid tumor.

Today, however, the most modern and progressive surgeons know that for the most part, only the growth itself needs to be removed, leaving your uterus and your childbearing options totally intact. The operation is called a myomectomy and it should always be the procedure of choice when nonmalignant fibroid tumors are disrupting your fertility.

HOW A MYOMECTOMY IS PERFORMED

Ths operation requires only one thin bikini incision right above your pubic bone and leaves only a minimal scar. Once inside, your surgeon makes a tiny slit into your uterus, lifts back the tissue, exposes your fibroid growths, and removes them at their base. Your incision is then stitched, and the operation is complete. Recovery time is four to five hospital days, with four to six weeks of home care.

WHY YOUR DOCTOR MIGHT SAY NO

As beneficial as myomectomies can be, not all doctors are qualified to perform them. For this reason, many physicians may not even inform you about this procedure. Some may try to scare you into having a hysterectomy by telling you that a myomectomy is a very bloody or risky operation. This objection is absolutely ungrounded. I have performed over a thousand myomectomies, and on only one occasion did a patient require a blood transfusion. Other fertility specialists who routinely perform this operation have had similar results. In fact, when done properly by an experienced myomectomy surgeon, the operation is one of the safest, most effective fertility-preserving procedures being performed today. You should give it prime consideration if you are diagnosed as having fibroid tumors that cannot be treated with medication.

WHAT YOUR DOCTOR SHOULD DO

Your doctor can help ensure a myomectomy's success and your safety, by taking the following precautions:

- ◆ A laser or an electrocautery knife should be used to "seal" cut blood vessels. This minimizes bleeding.
- ◆ A tourniquet should be placed around your uterus during the operation. This also cuts blood loss significantly.
- ◆ The drug petressin should be injected into the uterus, and an intravenous solution of the drug oxytocin should be used during the operation to minimize bleeding.
- ◆ Dextran 70, a highly viscous solution, should be injected into the abdomen, and the medication hydrocortisone should be given both intra-abdominally during the operation and intravenously for a few days following surgery to prevent the formation of abdominal adhesions, the scar tissue that can cause infertility.
- ◆ Antibiotics should be administered after surgery to guard against postoperative infection.

IF YOU DECIDE ON SURGERY: WHAT YOU NEED TO KNOW

If your doctor suggests that fertility surgery will help you, *you* must play an active, aggressive role in making that decision. The best way to do that is not only to find out as much as you can about your specific problem, but also to familiarize yourself with some of the specifics of the operation, as well as with some of the practical aspects of fertility surgery in general. Remember to solicit the following information from your doctor *well before* you schedule a surgery:

1. *The complete recovery time of your operation.* This includes any time spent in the hospital or office, as well as convalescing time at home.
2. *The rate of pregnancy after surgery.* While some fertility operations are genuinely worthwhile, others produce no significant results. Here are the success rates for pregnancy following some of the most common surgeries:

   - ◆ Salpingostomy: up to 39 percent
   - ◆ Fimbrioplasty: up to 67 percent
   - ◆ Tubal reimplantation: up to 32 percent
   - ◆ Anastomosis: up to 64 percent

3. *Your doctor's surgical qualifications.*

   ◆ How many fertility-related procedures has your physician performed, and particularly how many of the one he or she will be administering to you?
   ◆ How long has your doctor been doing fertility surgery?
   ◆ What precautions does your doctor plan to take to minimize the threat of postoperative complications and to hasten recovery time?
   ◆ What has been your doctor's success rate for pregnancies resulting from his operations?

   You have every right to know the answers to these questions, and if your doctor refuses to provide you with this information, seek help elsewhere.

4. *The total cost of your operation, including follow-up visits, and how much your insurance will cover.* Insurance plans vary greatly, so don't assume that every medical procedure is automatically covered by your policy. Some fertility treatments are not covered at all, while others are covered in full. Your doctor should have this information. If he or she does not, contact your insurance company, and get their reply in writing.

5. *Where the surgery will be performed, and the type of staff that will be caring for you.* This is vitally important if your doctor will be performing your surgery on an outpatient basis. Since all surgery requires at least two to three hours recovery time in the office or clinic in which it is performed, you need to know

   ◆ Are there qualified surgical and recovery room personnel, that is, are they experienced, trained, and certified, including board-certified anesthesiologists and registered nurses?
   ◆ Is the recovery room equipped to handle any medical emergencies that might arise from your operation?
   ◆ Does the clinic or hospital your doctor utilizes have a safe reputation? Ask for the names of patients who have had similar operations in the same facility, and question them on the care they received.

SOME FINAL ADVICE: KNOW ALL YOUR OPTIONS

Fertility surgery has come a long way in just the past five years, but as beneficial as these operations can be, they are not right for every woman. Sometimes surgery causes extensive scar tissue and even adhesions, for example, and you could end up with more fertility problems *after* your operation. A number of patients have come to me, frustrated and angry, as well as infertile, after their previous doctors had talked them into operations they never should have had.

WHEN SHOULD YOU THINK TWICE
ABOUT FERTILITY SURGERY?

If any of these conditions exist, an operation might not help you:

- Fallopian tubes that are severely blocked or damaged due either to a severe case of PID or to the occurrence of several cases over time
- Deeply imbedded scar tissue or adhesions on your ovaries or especially in your fallopian tubes
- Extensive endometriosis that has caused severe tubal and/or other organ damage, as well as excessive adhesions, all of which would be too difficult to repair surgically
- Extensive tubal or uterine damage due to previous surgery
- Tubal damage due to ectopic pregnacy

BE PRUDENT—BUT DON'T LOSE HOPE!

I tell you all this not to scare or dissuade you, only to help you decide wisely. Always get a second opinion—and if need be, a third—before making up your mind about having an operation.

In addition, keep in mind the many other pregnancy options, including the full array of laboratory-aided conceptions described in the final chapters of this book. Sometimes they can be a faster, easier, and even safer way to get pregnant than undergoing one or more surgical procedures.

· 17 ·

WHEN HE'S THE REASON YOU CAN'T CONCEIVE

The Newest Treatments for Male Infertility

Statistics now confirm what many fertility specialists have known for a long time—that almost half of all couples' fertility problems are male-related. I have certainly found this to be true in my own practice, where the number of female patients whose partners have reproductive problems has risen significantly in just the past few years.

Although there are a variety of different factors capable of affecting a man's fertility, the underlying cause is always sperm-related. For this reason, the very best and fastest way to determine if indeed your partner has a problem is a sperm count, which is actually an analysis of *several* factors related to fertility:

- *Number of sperm.* If the amount of sperm your partner manufactures is low (under 20 million sperm per milliliter), then chances for conception drop dramatically. If sperm count drops low enough, almost no chance for natural fertilization exists.
- *Sperm quality.* This refers to the percentage of *good* sperm your partner manufactures. A high sperm count means nothing if the percentage of healthy sperm is not also high. Unhealthy sperm (those that are deformed as a result of disease, a manufacturing defect, or a chromosomal abnormality) are usually too weak either to fertilize an egg or to bring about a successful conception

◆ *Sperm motility*. This describes the ability of sperm to reach your egg. If sperm motility is poor, then fertility will suffer. This condition often coexists with poor sperm quality.

Important note: Because all three factors can easily be influenced by bacterial infections, cultures should always be taken at the same time as a sperm count. This includes a check for infections to which your partner has been knowingly exposed and/or for which he is experiencing symptoms, as well as a check for any of the silent bacteria linked to infertility, such as chlamydia or T-mycoplasma.

If any infections are found, you, as well as your partner, must receive immediate treatment with antibiotics, as described in Chapter Four.

GOOD SPERM, BAD SPERM— WHAT DOES IT MEAN?

Although in some instances the results of a sperm count will be conclusive, with a clearly identifiable deficiency, at other times results may not be so easy to interpret. In fact, I have sometimes found that even two men with *identical* test results may not have equal success in conceiving a child. Why? Most often, your partner's fertility can be dependent on factors present in *your* body:

◆ If your reproductive system is *very* healthy and your partner has a borderline or low sperm count, conception can occur. Because your system presents no barriers, the few good sperm your partner does have, have a very good chance of reaching your egg.

◆ If, however, you have even a slight defect in your reproductive system (irregular ovulation, mild endometriosis, or a hostile vaginal environment, for example) then even a moderate sperm count can be too deficient to bring about a conception.

The status of each partner's fertility is so interdependent that most conception problems actually rest with the man and woman simultaneously. For this reason it's vital that your partner's sperm be analyzed *not* independently, but as an adjunct to *your* fertility.

IF SPERM IS BAD: THE NEXT STEP

A preliminary sperm count and bacterial culture can usually be taken by the same fertility specialist or clinic treating you. However, if the results indicate a problem, your partner should consider further testing with one of two types of male fertility specialists:

- *Urologist:* The male counterpart of your gynecologist, this specialist should be board-certified in urology (a broad category that covers disorders of the kidneys, urinary tract, bladder, and male reproductive organs). Additional training in reproductive endocrinology is a plus.
- *Andrologist.* These are scientists who study male reproduction. Most often they have a Ph.D. rather than an M.D. degree, with a specialty in biochemistry, endocrinology, or physiology. Frequently andrologists and/or embryologists are the laboratory specialists who direct the sperm procedures for fertility clinics.

THE MALE FERTILITY EXAM

Assuming sperm analysis and bacterial cultures have already taken place, a male fertility specialist will proceed with a physical exam beginning with the abdominal region and concentrate diagnostic efforts on the organs of the reproductive system:

- The penis
- The testicles
- Scrotal sac
- The vas deferens
- The rectum

The doctor will be looking for abnormalities in the shape, size, or tactile feel of these organs, as well as any skin eruptions, discolorations, or discharges. Most important, he or she will try to ascertain if there are any blockages anywhere in the reproductive tract, including any lumps, tumors, or cysts.

HOT TESTICLES: ONE CAUSE OF INFERTILITY

In addition the doctor should also make a point of checking for a condition called varicocele, which occurs when a vein outside the scrotum becomes dilated and enlarged (similar to varicose veins in the legs), allowing blood to pool in the testicles. This causes their temperature to rise and remain elevated, and as we've noted, when the temperature of the testicles rises too high, sperm production and motility can drop dramatically.

Responsible for up to 30 to 40 percent of male infertility, varicocele can begin as early as puberty, although many men do not experience its total impact until they are well into their thirties or even forties and may have even fathered one or more children.

However, it's also important to bear in mind that up to 15 percent of *all* men have varicocele, and many do not suffer its fertility-related consequences.

VARICOCELE REPAIR

In the event that a varicocele is diagnosed, immediate treatment via a simple surgical procedure is often recommended. Most men will experience improved sperm function right away, and in many instances complete fertility is restored.

The three major forms of repairing varicocele are traditional surgery, microsurgery, and a new procedure called a balloon occlusion, in which tiny implants help stop the flow of excess blood into the testicles. Each procedure has its own pros and cons, and your partner's doctor should advise him on the method that might be right for him.

THE VARICOCELE HOAX:
HOW TO AVOID UNNECESSARY SURGERY

Although varicocele repair can often greatly improve a man's fertility, this operation is somewhat *overrecommended*. In fact, unscrupulous doctors routinely recommend varicocele surgery when they diagnose minor, very tiny varicose veins that have little effect on sperm count and even when no problem exists. For this reason, I caution a man not to be persuaded into having this surgery unless there are clear-cut indications that the dilated veins are large enough to cause excess testicle heat.

As in the case of any operation, a man should get a second or even a third opinion if varicocele repair is recommended.

THE TESTICLE COOLER: A CONTROVERSIAL NEW
TREATMENT

In addition to the surgical options for correcting varicocele, a new device, aptly called a testicle cooler, is being used not only for this condition, but for any congenital vascular problem that can cause the temperature of a man's testicles to rise too high. Technically called a testicular hypothermia device, it works through the evaporation of water from the surface of the scrotum, reducing its temperature. A testicle cooler looks somewhat like a jock strap from which long, thin tubes have been extended. They're attached to a fluid reservoir (usually a small container that hooks onto a belt around the waist) that also acts as a pump. The water circulates through the tubes and keeps the testicles cool.

Still somewhat primitive, the device must be worn daily whenever a man is awake and clothed. The water reservoir must be filled every six hours. The unit can be removed for bathing, sleeping, and sex. Most users claim it is fairly comfortable and easy to conceal. However, it often must be used for prolonged periods of time before positive effects are seen.

MORE TESTS FOR MALE INFERTILITY

In addition to the physical exam, the reason for an abnormal sperm count can also often be revealed in one or more of the following blood tests:

- ♦ *T3 and T4 Thyroid Function Tests.* When thyroid function is low (hypothyroidism) sperm production can become so sluggish that it nearly comes to a complete halt. In most instances thyroid medication can restore the function of this important gland and in the process help return sperm production and count to normal.
- ♦ *FSH and LH.* The same brain hormones that affect a woman's egg production also affect sperm production in your partner. If levels drop too low, a sperm deficiency can develop.

    Treatment with fertility drugs like clomiphene citrate (Clomid), menotropins (Pergonal), and hCG (described in Chapter Eighteen) can help restore sperm count and increase fertility.
- ♦ *Testosterone.* Deficiencies in this hormone can be an indication of a biochemical imbalance or problems within the testicles themselves. If testosterone is low, additional diagnostic procedures, including a testicle biopsy (you'll read about this in a moment), may be needed.

WHEN LOW SPERM COUNT IS ONLY TEMPORARY

Sometimes low sperm count is temporary, brought on by any number of passing factors in a man's life:

- ♦ Colds, the flu, a virus
- ♦ Any infection that causes his white blood cell count to rise—an abscessed tooth, an infected finger or toe, etc.
- ♦ Poor nutrition, especially deficiencies in zinc, vitamin C, and the B-complex vitamins
- ♦ Overuse of cigarettes, alcohol, or any use of street drugs
- ♦ Certain medications, especially those used to treat high blood pressure or ulcers
- ♦ Stress
- ♦ Lack of sleep

If any of these conditions exist at the time a man has his sperm checked, he should notify his doctor. Before seeking further fertility treatment, he should have at least one more sperm count taken when these conditions do not exist.

WHEN SPERM CAN'T LEAVE A MAN'S BODY: ANOTHER CAUSE OF INFERTILITY

If the quality of your partner's sperm is good but the overall amount present in each ejaculation is low, his problem may be one of sperm transport. A blockage somewhere in his reproductive tract, most often the vas deferens (the hollow tube that transports sperm from the testicles to the penis), is keeping some or all of his sperm from leaving his body. To check for this problem, one of three diagnostic procedures can be used:

- *Fluid aspiration.* Here, fluid taken directly from the vas deferens is checked for sperm. If sperm are found residing in the fluid, it is likely blockage exists that is keeping them from leaving the body.
- *The saline test.* A harmless saline (salt) solution is injected into the vas. If it flows easily, it is likely that no blockages exist. If it does not flow easily, the physician can insert an ultrathin catheter into the vas and slowly move it along the inside. If the catheter meets resistance, it usually means a blockage exists.
- *The vasogram.* In the event that either of these tests proves inconclusive, your partner's doctor may want to perform a vasogram, a kind of male fertility x-ray. Similar to a hysterosalpingogram used to find blockages in your fallopian tubes, in this test a high-contrast dye is injected into the vas deferens through a small incision in the scrotal sac. Using x-rays to monitor the flow of the dye, the specialist can determine where a blockage might lie.

Important warning about vasograms: Although an extremely effective diagnostic procedure, unless performed by a highly trained, experienced vasogram specialist, this test can harm a man's fertility by damaging the delicate tubal ducts leading to the vas, a problem that must be remedied via immediate emergency surgery. For this reason, this test should only be given in extreme cases.

VAS SURGERY: HOW TO RESTORE FERTILITY

Should a blockage in the vas deferens (the cause of 10 percent of male fertility problems) be discovered, microsurgery can help. Various operations to open blocked areas of the vas and remove obstructions often restore fertility in just a few months.

LACK OF SEMEN: ANOTHER CAUSE OF INFERTILITY

In addition to blockages in the vas deferens, your partner may simply not have enough ejaculatory fluid to adequately carry his sperm through his body and into yours. To ascertain if this problem exists, your partner can have a sugar test, which measures the effectiveness of the seminal vesicles, the glands located on the vas deferens that help supply ejaculatory fluid.

Since all fluids flowing from the seminal vesicles leave the gland in the same fashion, it's necessary to test for only one in order to verify their function. Fructose (fruit sugar) is one of those fluids, and it can be easily tested.

The test requires that your partner masturbate at least one ejaculation into a sterile container. If no sugar is found in the semen, then a defect in the seminal vesicles might exist, most often a blockage in the ducts leading to the vas deferens. If this is found to be true, microsurgery to open the ducts can often restore fertility.

THE BLOCKED EPIDIDYMIS: WHEN SPERM CAN'T MOVE

Perhaps the ultimate transport problem exists when sperm simply cannot leave the epididymis, which is located just atop the testicles, where sperm matures and learns to *swim*. Sperm leave the epididymis through tiny ducts connected to the vas deferens. When, due to infection (primarily caused by STDs), those ducts become blocked, some or even all sperm can be kept from leaving.

If this condition is diagnosed, microsurgery can help. The operation is successful about 50 percent of the time, in terms of restoring sperm count, but only about 20 percent of the patients regain their fertility. Why? When an epididymis is surgically repaired, only the ducts are opened. If the infection has affected the organ itself, the sperm will pass through the epididymis but will not acquire the swimming skills necessary to navigate through a woman's reproductive system and reach her egg.

The orange dye test, which was developed to measure levels of DNA (the substance that makes up chromosomes) in sperm, can be used to learn whether sperm motility has been compromised. When levels are low, sperm is clinically dead; movement is slow and erratic. By measuring levels of DNA, this test can detect a sperm's potential for moving quickly and effortlessly through your cervical mucus and down your fallopian tubes.

Even if no sperm motility is found, a man may still be able to father a child via artificial insemination and/or in vitro fertilization, two laboratory-aided conceptions where navigational ability of sperm is not necessary. (They're described in Chapters Nineteen and Twenty).

CAN YOUR PARTNER'S SPERM FERTILIZE YOUR EGG? HOW TO TELL

Before conception can occur, sperm must first penetrate the multilayered coating of your egg's outer shell. In order to accomplish this, the head of each sperm (called the acrosome) contains a packet of enzymes to help break down the coating of your egg; these are released as soon as contact is made. If the head of a sperm or the enzymes are in any way deficient, infertility can be the result.

To test its penetrating ability, sperm is placed in a test tube containing eggs. Because hamster eggs are very similar to human eggs, they are often used for this test; hence the name, hamster egg test. If, after twenty-four hours, the sperm does not penetrate the hamster eggs (a negative result), fertilization of human eggs would not be likely to occur, either.

IMPORTANT NOTE

Up to 10 percent of men who have a negative hamster egg test result (indicating a penetration problem) are successful with laboratory-aided conceptions. Conversely, some men with positive test results (indicating no sperm penetration problem) cannot fertilize a *human* egg, either naturally or in the lab. Finally, because the medium used in the tests can affect the outcome, and because media can vary from lab to lab, test results can often vary with the same sperm sample. In addition, sperm penetration ability can vary from day to day, so one hamster test is never considered a definitive diagnostic assessment.

THE ULTIMATE TEST OF MALE FERTILITY

Perhaps the most accurate of all fertility tests is one that mixes your partner's sperm with your egg in a laboratory to see if fertilization can occur. It is most often used in conjunction with in vitro fertilization and the GIFT procedure (two types of laboratory-aided conceptions you'll read about later) as a way of predicting the success of these procedures.

THE TESTICLE BIOPSY: WHEN IT'S NECESSARY—WHEN IT'S NOT

In a very small percentage of men, sperm count is zero. If a physical exam fails to reveal a blockage and if testicles appear small and soft and blood levels of FSH are high (more than twice the normal reading), a testicle biospy may be necessary to determine the source of the problem.

Much like an ovarian biopsy, this procedure involves the surgical removal of a small sample of tissue from inside the testicles, which is then examined under a microscope for evidence that sperm is being produced. It is usually done on an outpatient basis, and the surgery itself requires no stitches. Normally a man can be back at work in just a day or two.

WHAT A BIOPSY CAN REVEAL

If the tissue sample taken during the biopsy shows that no sperm is present, the testicles are assumed to be nonfunctioning. There is generally no treatment for this condition. If sperm *are* found in the tissue but are absent from the ejaculate, the problem probably lies in the transport system, and your partner should be reexamined for blockages or other related problems.

WARNING: DON'T HAVE A TESTICLE BIOPSY WITHOUT HAVING THIS TEST

Sometimes a deficiency in your partner's pituitary gland prevents his testicles from receiving the go-signal to manufacture sperm. This condition, called hypogonadotropic hypogonadism, is also characterized by a zero sperm count. For this reason, a man should never be subjected to a testicle biopsy *until* he has been tested at least once, with a follow-up verification test about thirty days later, for levels of FSH and LH, the two sperm-producing triggers supplied by the pituitary.

If levels are abnormal or even borderline suspect, a man should be treated with fertility drugs before undergoing a testicle biopsy.

FERTILITY ANTIBODIES: WHEN A MAN'S BODY TURNS AGAINST HIM

One of the latest discoveries to surface in the field of reproductive medicine is the link between the immune system and infertility. In some individuals a curious problem causes the immune system to go awry and begin manufacturing sperm antibodies, the same kind that are used to fight disease. In this instance, however, the antibodies fight—and kill—sperm. When *your* system manufactures these antibodies, they most often appear in your cervical mucus and attack sperm as they enter your vagina. A far more serious condition exists when a man's body makes the antibodies that damage or destroy his own sperm before it gets to you.

HOW A MAN CAN SAVE HIS SPERM

For men who manufacture sperm antibodies, steroid medications like prednisone or dexamethasone can sometimes help. However, because treatment often requires high dosages, which invites a host of potentially serious complications, these drugs should not be commonly prescribed.

Another, far more popular way of coping with sperm antibodies is conception via artificial intrauterine insemination. In preparation for this process, sperm is *washed*. Although this cannot remove antibodies, it does serve to extract the best-quality sperm and make them available for fertilization. A full explanation of sperm washing is included in Chapter Nineteen.

RESTORING MALE FERTILITY: REVERSING A VASECTOMY

One of the most important male fertility operations is the reversing of a vasectomy, the male birth-control procedure. In a vasectomy a section of vas deferens closest to the epididymis (about an inch) is cut, and the ends sealed with stitches, heat, or clips. This keeps sperm from passing through a man's reproductive tract; instead of leaving his body during an ejaculation, it simply dies and disintegrates. The operation to reverse a vasectomy is in some ways similar to the procedure to reverse a voluntary tubal sterilization in your body. It involves opening the area of the vas that was surgically closed and reattaching the cut ends.

If your partner is thinking about reversing a vasectomy, he should be aware that the longer he waits, the lower his chances for a successful reversal:

- Men who have had vasectomies ten years or longer have less than a 40 percent chance of conceiving after a vasectomy reversal.
- Men who have had vasectomies less than ten years have about a 90 percent chance of ejaculating sperm after a vasectomy reversal.

IMPORTANT WARNING: WHEN A VASECTOMY REVERSAL CAUSES A SPERM ALLERGY

In some men, a vasectomy can cause the production of sperm antibodies, a problem that doesn't appear until a reversal surgery is performed. In fact, up to two-thirds of all men who have vasectomies develop antibodies that can interfere with sperm motility and fertilization upon reversal.

WHEN YOUR PARTNER CAN'T EJACULATE: WHAT CAN HELP

In a very small percentage of men, a zero sperm count is an indication of a condition called retrograde ejaculation. Most commonly due to nerve damage that results from diabetes, this condition occurs when the muscle used to close the bladder right before orgasm and ejaculation (keeping passing sperm from taking the wrong turn on the way to the penis) does not function as it normally should. As a result, semen is routed into a man's bladder rather than down his urethra and out his penis. The easiest way to test for this problem is to simply analyze a man's urine after he ejaculates. If sperm are present, retrograde ejaculation is likely to be occurring

---

TREATMENT FOR EJACULATION PROBLEMS

Currently the only treatment for retrograde ejaculation is a series of drugs, similar to decongestants, that cause a constrictive or tightening effect on the opening of the bladder.

Barring that solution, the only possibility left is artificial insemination, the sperm being extracted directly from the bladder via a catheter. Because urine is highly acidic and normally kills sperm, the catheter contains a buffer solution to provide the alkaline environment sperm need to survive. (The man can also drink a highly alkaline solution like baking soda a few hours before ejaculating. This will help preserve sperm in the urine.) Because, however, sperm that have been in the bladder are generally of poor quality, even with these procedures, pregnancy is only achieved about 10 percent of the time.

OVERCOMING IMPOTENCE: HOW YOU CAN STILL CONCEIVE

One of the most emotionally and physically devastating causes of infertility is impotence. Sperm count and motility can be perfect, but unless a man can have an erection, he cannot naturally deposit his sperm in his partner's body.

Currently, 10 percent of all male infertility is due to impotence, and there is an increasing number of impotent men in their prime reproductive years, between ages twenty-five and thirty-five. Once thought to be a condition associated with aging, the latest research shows that almost as many young men lose their ability to get an erection as men who are past age fifty.

In the not too distant past it was believed that nearly all causes of impotence were psychological. Today, we know that not to be true. While impotence can be due to emotional problems, including depression, anxiety, and fear, in most cases its cause is rooted in a physiological problem.

IMPOTENCE: THE MOST COMMON CAUSES AND THE FASTEST CURES

1. *Cause: environmental factors.* Cocaine, marijuana, caffeine, alcohol, and cigarettes constrict blood supply to the penis necessary for an erection.
   Cure: Discontinuing use of these substances should reverse impotency within a few weeks.
2. *Cause: medications.* Drugs used to treat high blood pressure, depression, and anxiety are especially detrimental.
   Cure: Substitute a different drug or discontinue treatment. In most cases impotence is reversed when drugs are stopped.
3. *Cause: increased prolactin levels.* Due to a tumor or other hormonal imbalances, increased prolactin levels result in low sex drive and impotence.
   Cure: The medication bromocriptine mesylate (Parlodel) lowers prolactin levels, shrinks tumors, and restores the ability to have an erection about 50 percent of the time.
4. *Cause: disease.* Especially harmful are diseases that reduce blood flow to the penis, such as diabetes or hardening of the arteries. In addition, conditions that can damage the nerves leading to the penis, such as stroke, spinal cord injuries, kidney disease, diabetes, or back injuries, can also cause impotence.
   Cure: Often proper management of the disease itself can reverse the impotency. When it can't, penile implants and electroejaculation devices can help (they're both discussed shortly).
5. *Cause: leaky veins.* Up to 20 percent of all cases of physiological impotence occur when a leaky vein inside the penis reduces the blood volume necessary to achieve and/or maintain an erection.
   Cure: Microsurgery. The leaky veins are tied off, keeping blood volume in the penis from dropping.

IF IMPOTENCE IS A PROBLEM, DON'T WAIT—GET HELP!

There is probably not a man alive who at some point in his life will not experience at least one temporary bout with impotence. In fact, the system that allows a man to get an erection is among the most vulnerable in the human body; sometimes even a case of simple exhaustion can affect both his sex drive and his ability to perform. Both, of course, affect his fertility.

However, for some men, impotence is not a passing incident, but a clinical problem. If your partner goes more than two weeks without being able to achieve an erection (with you, during solo masturbation, or unconsciously while asleep) and if none of the environmental factors linked to this problem is present, then he must see his doctor.

In most cases, treating or eliminating the physical factor will result in a full restoration of potency within only a few weeks. If no physical causes can be found, sex therapy can be successful in overcoming impotence up to 80 percent of the time.

PREMATURE EJACULATION AND FERTILITY

In addition to not being able to get an erection, impotency can also manifest itself in a condition called premature ejaculation syndrome, in which a man can get an erection, but he can't maintain it long enough to deposit sperm into your vagina. In many cases, psychological counseling can help overcome this problem. If it can't, you can still achieve a pregnancy via artificial insemination. In fact, even if your man has a soft or semisoft penis, he can still ejaculate via masturbation. In some instances your doctor can teach him how to aspirate the sperm into a syringe and inject it into your vagina in the privacy of your bedroom.

MORE GOOD NEWS: NEW WAYS FOR AN IMPOTENT MAN TO FATHER A CHILD!

Although most men find a cure for their potency problems, some need additional help to conceive. One type of aid is the penile prosthesis, or implant, a relatively new way to assist a man in obtaining and maintaining an erection. Currently, two different types of penile implants are available, those that are rigid and those that are inflatable. Both involve a simple installation operation.

- ◆ Rigid devices involve implanting silicone rods that, though bendable, remain erect inside the penis all the time.
- ◆ Inflatable devices also involve implanting a rod but have the added convenience of a pump reservoir that allows a man to control erections by inflating or deflating the implant.

Since impotency does not affect sperm manufacture or quality, once the erection problem is solved, you should be able to conceive naturally.

THE NEW MALE FERTILITY TECHNOLOGY

Currently it is estimated that 250,000 men in the United States are unable to conceive a child due to a spinal cord injury that has inhibited their ability to ejaculate. Tens of thousands more with diseases like multiple sclerosis, diabetes, and testicular cancer have the same problem.

Now, thanks to a brand-new fertility technology, even a man who cannot ejaculate can still father a child with the assistance of electro-ejaculation, a technique used to obtain sperm. Placing a probe inside the man's rectum, a technician delivers a mild surge of current that reaches the prostrate gland, causing a series of stimulating motions that usually produce an erection and ejaculation within four minutes. The sperm is later artificially inseminated into the woman.

Although experiments with electroejaculation began as early as 1948, it wasn't until just as few years ago that this technique, and the insemination procedures it requires, were perfected. Currently many fertility clinics around the country are offering new hope to infertile couples via this therapy.

DRUGS, POTIONS, AND OTHER POTENCY CURES: WHAT WORKS AND WHAT DOESN'T

Perhaps the most widespread misconceptions in the world of medicine surround the medications and drugs purported to increase a man's potency. Nearly every week a patient brings to my attention a magazine or mail-order advertisement boasting the ability of various products to stimulate a man's sexual prowess. Some are even billed as fertility drugs, claiming to increase sperm production as well as potency.

Do these products work? Most often they do not. There are, however, a *few* medications that have provided some help for some men:

- *Papaverine,* a chemical derived from the papaya plant, causes blood vessels to dilate throughout the body and can increase blood flow to the penis. If impotence is caused by a constriction of blood vessels or by nerve damage to these vessels, by injecting this drug directly into his penis prior to having sex, a man can stimulate an erection.
- *Prostaglandin E1,* a chemical made naturally in the body, can also work to stimulate vessel dilation and blood flow to the penis when injected just prior to sex.
- *Yocon* (generic name, yohimbine hydrochloride), a prescription drug, works by constricting the blood vessels in the penis, helping to keep blood from escaping. This keeps penile blood volume high in men who can get an erection but can't maintain it.

A FINAL WORD

The treatment of male fertility has been advancing rapidly in the past few years, and a great deal of research continues, giving men with fertility problems greater hope than ever for fathering a child. However, it's imperative that a man actively seek help the moment a problem is suspected. If diagnosed early on, treatment is usually fast and easy and can bring about a healthy conception a month or two later.

Because, however, many men still find it difficult to accept the possibility that they have a fertility problem, it's imperative that you encourage your partner, gently but firmly, to play an active role in conception by having at least a preliminary fertility workup at the same time as yours.

In some instances, when your BBT and other ovulatory signs are normal, and especially if you have been pregnant with another partner before, he should be tested *before* you receive any extensive workups.

· 18 ·

SUPEROVULATION AND OTHER NEW WAYS TO A FASTER, EASIER CONCEPTION

Although many steps and functions are involved in making a baby, for you, the core of your fertility lies in your ability to manufacture and release good eggs. By "good" I mean eggs that begin developing at the start of your cycle, grow to full maturity, release enough estrogen to signal ovulation, and finally, pop from their shell and ovulate into your fallopian tube at the precise point that fertilization is optimum.

For most women, this egg-making process progresses in a natural, orderly pattern, one that does lead to conception. However, for some the process doesn't go quite this smoothly. Deficiencies in the hormones needed to stimulate egg growth, development, or release can make conception difficult. If hormone levels drop low enough, complete biochemical infertility can result.

The newest and perhaps the most successful way to correct these egg-related problems is with fertility drugs, medications that stimulate or supplement the production of one or more of the following hormones necessary for the development and release of healthy eggs:

 • Follicle-stimulating hormone (FSH)
 • Luteinizing hormone (LH)
 • Gonadotropin-releasing hormone (GnRH)

Often two or three cycles using fertility drugs are all you need to conceive naturally. In fact, I have had many infertile patients who were able to get pregnant after taking one or two of these medications for as little as sixty days!

SUPEROVULATION: A NEW WAY TO USE FERTILITY DRUGS

One of the newest ways to use fertility drugs is called superovulation. In this treatment women with no significant egg-related problems are given one or more of these medications in order to help increase both the amount and the quality of the eggs they produce. This can be especially helpful if your partner has a low sperm count, since the healthier your eggs are, the better the chances for a healthy fertilization. Superovulation also improves chances for success with artificial insemination and in vitro fertilization. Again, the healthier your eggs, and in the case of in vitro the more eggs you have, the better the chances for fertilization.

HOW SUPEROVULATION HELPS YOU HAVE A BETTER PREGNANCY

In addition to increasing your egg-making potential, I have found fertility drugs to be a great way to achieve a healthier pregnancy overall. Studies show that superovulation can actually decrease your risk of miscarriage and premature labor and help promote a healthier implantation. How?

- Fertility drugs help you make more eggs, which in turn means more estrogen. This can help increase the quality of your cervical mucus (necessary for a good vaginal or cervical insemination) and lead to a thicker endometrial lining, which aids implantation.
- In addition, more eggs also means more corpus luteum, the material that constitutes the shells of your eggs and produces progesterone in the second half of your menstrual cycle. High progesterone can help prevent miscarriage by quieting uterine cramping and building a strong endometrial lining. This promotes a healthy implantation and helps to provide your baby with adequate nourishment right from the start of your pregnancy.

For these reasons I often use fertility drugs to treat patients whose family or personal health history indicates they may be susceptible to premature labor or pregnancy loss. Although the chances for multiple birth increase by about 25 percent when superovulation is used (due to the effects of the fertility drugs), most often the result is twins.

ARE FERTILITY DRUGS SAFE?

As beneficial as these medications have proved to be, they are probably the most misunderstood drugs being used today. For some couples, even the mere mention of the term conjures up scary images of everything from Siamese twins to quintuplets to deformed babies. These fears have absolutely no basis in reality.

In fact, I can tell you, based on clinical studies and on my personal experience, having prescribed fertility drugs for hundreds of patients, most, if not all, of the preparations your doctor uses to stimulate your fertility are among the safest medications available. This is because most were developed to simulate *natural* functions of your body. Many are in fact natural supplements of chemicals your body already manufactures every day—or would manufacture if it were working perfectly.

And contrary to a common misconception, fertility drugs are not directly involved with the fertilization process: they are out of your system before conception takes place. This is why they generally have no residual effects on your baby.

THE MOST COMMON FERTILITY DRUGS AND HOW THEY WORK

Although technically any drug that helps you get pregnant can be called a fertility medication, there are currently five treatments, all of them working directly on egg production and release, that most specialists classify as fertility drugs. To help you understand a little more about each of them, I have prepared this special guide. It features some of the information you need to know if your doctor prescribes these drugs.

The medications are listed in alphabetical order, so their place in the guide holds no special significance in terms of usefulness or safety.

DRUG: CLOMIPHENE CITRATE
BRAND NAME: CLOMID, SEROPHENE

What You Need to Know

Most often prescribed to help encourage ovulation, this drug helps you manufacture stronger, healthier eggs.

It is administered in tablet form, and most women who take this drug have about an 80 percent chance of ovulating and a 50 percent chance of getting pregnant within six months of treatment. The risk of multiple births is only minimally higher than in natural pregnancy.

Possible side effects can include hot flashes, abdominal bloating, nausea, breast tenderness, fatigue, nervous tension, visual disturbances and ovarian enlargement.

This drug can also affect the production of cervical mucus while it is being taken, decreasing the amount and making what is available so thick it can actually keep sperm from reaching your egg.

To help overcome this problem, many of my patients have found that taking several daily doses of an expectorant cough medicine like Robitussin helps. It works by thinning all mucus secretions in the body and can overcome the vaginal dryness that clomiphene citrate sometimes causes. To promote production of even more cervical mucus, your doctor may occasionally prescribe small amounts of estrogen to be taken simultaneously with clomiphene citrate.

DRUG: GONADOTROPIN-RELEASING HORMONE (GnRH)
BRAND NAME: NONE

What You Need to Know

This drug increases your fertility by supplementing levels of GnRH, the hormone that helps trigger the entire egg production process. It is usually given when your body does not manufacture enough on its own.

It can be especially helpful if you suffer an irregular menstrual cycle and/or irregular ovulation after discontinuing birth control pills or if you have a lack of progesterone in the second half of your menstrual cycle (called a luteal phase defect). It can also stimulate menstrual activity in female athletes when excessive exercise has caused a sharp decline in the production of all reproductive hormones.

The pregnancy rate for GnRH therapy is two out of three, within four months, and there is almost no risk of an increase in multiple births.

GnRH is relatively free of any significant side effects. It is administered by injection every other day or via an infusion pump. In the latter, a thin needle is implanted under your skin or inserted directly into your vein like an I.V. The needle is attached to a catheter connected to a small box that is worn around the waist. This box delivers a spurt of GnRH every ninety minutes, mimicking almost exactly the way your body would deliver this hormone.

DRUG: HUMAN CHORIONIC GONADOTROPIN (hCG)
BRAND NAME: PROFASI, PREGNYL, A.P.L.

What You Need to Know

Under normal circumstances, LH is the hormone that signals ovulation. If it is in short supply, ovulation does not occur. An LH deficiency can be overcome by using hCG, a hormone that is normally manufactured by your baby's placenta after you are already pregnant. Because it is similar in structure to LH, it also works to trigger egg release.

In addition, hCG is thought to help initiate the production of pro- gesterone directly after ovulation, so it can also be used to treat a luteal phase defect, in which progesterone is in short supply in the second half of the menstrual cycle. This can help protect you against miscarriage.

This drug is administered via injection, usually given just once in your cycle, immediately prior to the time at which you would normally ovulate. An ultrasonogram of your eggs can determine their maturity and help predict the exact day hCG should be administered.

Possible side effects for hCG include headaches, irritability, restless- ness, depression, fatigue, edema, and hyperstimulation (see next entry).

Pure LH, in the form of a drug called Factrel, is currently being tested and may be available in the near future for treatment purposes.

DRUG: MENOTROPINS
BRAND NAME: PERGONAL

What You Need to Know

This drug increases fertility by helping you release more mature eggs and ensuring that ovulation occurs. It works by supplementing your body with FSH and LH, the hormones that initiate egg production and release. Rather than stimulating your own system to make more of these hormones, Pergonal supplies them directly to your ovaries, via your bloodstream.

It is the primary drug used for superovulation and to prepare your body for in vitro fertilization and artificial insemination. Pergonal is administered by daily injection into your buttocks. It induces ovulation in about 90 percent of the women who take it, and about 50 percent become pregnant within six months.

As effective and safe as Pergonal is, it can lead to a condition called hyperstimulation, in which you manufacture so many eggs that your ovaries can enlarge to painful proportions, a situation that even an expert fertility specialist cannot always control. In some instances overstimula- tion can become so severe that hospitalization may be required to admin- ister intravenous solution and monitor your body's electrolyte balance. Milder cases of hyperstimulation can be treated on a outpatient basis.

To help prevent hyperstimulation, your doctor should take sonograms of your ovaries and an E2 estrogen blood test every day or every other day. Both these tests can help indicate if eggs are growing too rapidly or too large. If they are, fertility medications should be immediately stopped and ovulation prevented by withholding your injection of hCG.

From 10 to 25 percent of births resulting from this drug are multiples, with the majority being twins.

DRUG: UROFOLLITROPIN
BRAND NAME: METRODIN

What You Need to Know

This drug is pure FSH, and it increases fertility when an excess of LH is present in your body. By rebalancing the delicate FSH–LH ratio, it helps ensure that you will make eggs and ovulate. I have also used this drug to rebalance FSH levels that are slightly elevated but still within the normal range. It can also work well for women who have not responded to treatment with either Clomid or Pergonal or with a combination regimen. It is administered in tablet form. It does cause an increased risk of multiple births, most commonly twins.

Possible side effects include ovarian enlargement and hyperstimulation syndrome (see Pergonal, above).

THE DRUGS THAT HELP FERTILITY DRUGS WORK

It is often difficult to judge how a given patient will react to fertility drugs. There is always the possibility that her body will receive too much stimulation, causing her hormone levels to rise too high, thus creating another type of imbalance problem, reducing rather than enhancing fertility. To keep this from happening, medications classified as agonists are used to shut down your body's natural production of hormones, allowing only the controlled amount supplied by the fertility drugs to circulate through your system. The two most commonly used for this purpose are leuprolide acetate (Lupron) and Nafarelin.

- *Lupron.* This drug is administered as an injection. While it is currently approved by the FDA only for use on prostatic cancer in men, it is widely used in fertility clinics in other parts of the world for the purposes described here. It is expected to be approved in the United States for this purpose shortly. One down point: it does not work for all women; the reasons remain unknown.
- *Nafarelin.* Currently available as a nasal spray, this drug has only been approved in the United States for the treatment of endometriosis. However, because it is used in fertility clinics worldwide, it is also expected to be approved in the United States as a fertility drug in the near future.

Generally there are no significant side effects for either drug when used in conjunction with other fertility medications.

AN IMPORTANT WARNING

One of the most beneficial aspects of all fertility drugs is that they can be used in so many different ways. By altering the dosage, the number of days the drug is taken, and, most important, the combination of drugs used, your doctor can arrive at the precise biochemical balance needed to help you achieve a safe and healthy conception. However, regardless of the treatment regimen used, it is extremely important that only a physician with experience and expertise in prescribing these drugs, one who is willing, moreover, to put the time and energy into daily monitoring and care, administer these medications. In the hands of such a specialist, these preparations are safe and highly effective. However, in the wrong hands, a number of serious, sometimes life-threatening complications can result.

For this reason, *never* accept fertility drugs from anyone other than a fertility specialist or a gynecologist/obstetrician who has been specially trained in this area. If you are not being monitored at least every other day (with a sonogram and estrogen blood tests) and especially if your doctor does not address any side effects you report having while using these medications, *stop your regimen immediately,* and find a specialist who can help you.

THE DRUGS THAT WORK ON SPECIFIC PROBLEMS

In addition to the medications that work on egg production and release, there are a number of other types of drugs that can increase your fertility by correcting the medical problems that directly affect your reproductive health. If you are diagnosed as infertile due to a specific disease or condition, it's possible that one or more of the following medications can help.

- ◆ *Corticosteroids, spironolactone.* These two categories of medication are used in the treatment of hyperandrogynism (an overproduction of the steroid hormones called androgens), as well as polycystic ovarian syndrome and antisperm antibodies in men and women. Their goal is to reduce the amount of androgens in your system and/or suppress the immune system.
- ◆ *Danazol (Danocrine).* This medication is used primarily in the treatment of endometriosis. It works by blocking the production of

estrogen in your body, without which endometrial lesions shrivel and die.

- *Estrogen.* When estrogen levels are low, mucus becomes thick and elastic, acting as a natural diaphragm, keeping sperm out instead of making it easier for them to enter. Available in pills or in patches worn on the skin, estrogen supplements increase fertility by encouraging the production of more and thinner cervical mucus, allowing for easier sperm transport.
- *Natural progesterone.* This is used primarily in the treatment of a luteal phase defect, a problem that can increase your risk of miscarriage and/or premature labor. The defeat develops when, for various reasons, your body does not manufacture enough progesterone in the second half of your menstrual cycle. Treatment is available in the form of an injection or as a vaginal suppository.
- *Bromocriptine mesylate (Parlodel).* This is used in the treatment of hyperprolactemia, a condition that inhibits egg production and can stop ovulation. It is characterized by the overproduction of the hormone prolactin, which can occur due to a malfunction in your pituitary gland, most often a benign tumor. A common symptom of this condition is leakage of breast milk even when you are not lactating. Parlodel works directly on your pituitary gland, inhibiting the production of prolactin and often shrinking the tumors that cause the excess.
- *Thyroid medication.* Since your thyroid helps to regulate the flow and timing of all reproductive (and other) hormones, when this gland works too fast or too slow, all other biochemicals respond accordingly. In the case of your reproductive hormones FSH and LH, a thyroid problem can mean eggs are not produced or released on time or even at all. Thyroid medications increase fertility by helping to regulate the function and timing of this important gland, returning your chemical time clock to normal.

THE NEW HORMONE THAT CAN AFFECT YOUR FERTILITY

One of the most recent discoveries made in reproductive medicine is the existence of a new hormone called activin. Researchers predict this biochemical may hold the key to a great number of infertility problems.

Although the full function of this hormone is not yet clear, in animal studies it was found that even in small amounts it led to a doubling of the number of eggs released. It has also shown evidence of reducing androgen levels and rebalancing a high LH–FSH ratio, associated with polycystic ovarian syndrome.

Activin has also been found to increase levels of progesterone and hCG and is now being considered as a remedy for recurring miscarriages due to a deficiency in these hormones. In men, activin seems to increase sperm production.

Although activin is available in limited supply, for experimental research use only, it is hoped that in the near future supplements of this hormone will be more widely available for infertility treatments.

WHEN MEN NEED FERTILITY DRUGS

Although male infertility has usually been associated with functional or structural problems, recent research has shown that the vast majority of problems occur due to hormonal disorders. Like a woman, a man needs the proper endocrine system interaction (in his case, among his hypothalamus, pituitary, and testicles) if he is to manufacture not only adequate amounts of sperm, but sperm of good quality.

Because the same brain hormones, FSH and LH, are involved in both your reproductive process and your partner's, sometimes men can benefit from the use of the same drugs that stimulate the production of these hormones in your body.

THE FERTILITY DRUGS FOR MEN

- ◆ Clomiphene citrate (Clomid, Serophene)
- ◆ Pergonal and hCG
- ◆ GnRH
- ◆ Bromocriptine mesylate
- ◆ Thyroid replacement medications

FERTILITY DRUGS AND LABORATORY-AIDED CONCEPTIONS

In addition to stimulating egg production for natural conception, fertility drugs are used in conjunction with the following laboratory-aided conceptions:

- ◆ Artificial insemination
- ◆ Intrauterine insemination
- ◆ In vitro fertilization
- ◆ The GIFT and ZIFT procedures

Although much higher doses are normally needed for this purpose, the goal is still the same: the production and maturation of healthy eggs. In fact, because these procedures require that you produce a multitude of eggs (to increase chances for fertilization), even if you are manufacturing them on your own, superovulation can be used to increase your chance for conception. (See the chapters that follow.)

FERTILITY DRUGS AND YOU: A COMMITMENT TO PREGNANCY

There is no doubt that fertility drugs can and will increase your ability to get pregnant. However, you, your partner, and your doctor *must* make a joint commitment to your pregnancy:

- Medications must be taken with unfailing accuracy. Timing is often crucial. Since many of these drugs are injected, your partner can be taught to administer the shot, saving you a trip to your doctor's office and allowing you a more flexible schedule.
- As with all drugs, you should become familiar with any and all side effects your medication can cause. Immediately report to your doctor any that occur. This is especially important in preventing hyperstimulation syndrome and/or in alerting your doctor to the need to decrease dosages to better help you conceive.
- You must make the required trips to your doctor for sonograms and blood tests. Missing even one scheduled session could have disastrous results—or at the very least keep you from getting pregnant.
- For the period during which you are taking the drugs, you must plan your social and your sexual life around your medication regimens. That means weekend trips or vacations must sometimes be postponed if they interfere in any way with your checkups. Sex must be timed with your medication to make optimum use of its fertility-increasing powers.
- Finally, you must resign yourself to the possibility of a multiple birth. Although not every couple who uses fertility drugs has more than one baby, the chances increase with the amount of drugs you take. Of course, if you have been infertile for a long time, multiples are a great way to *catch up* with your family planning.

It's also important that you not become discouraged if a pregnancy does not result right away. Many different regimens and combinations of fertility drugs are available, and it may take a while to strike the right recipe for you. With patience, and with the skill of a good specialist, fertility drugs have answered the prayer for motherhood for tens of thousands of women worldwide. They can be your answer, too.

• 19 •

THE NEW ARTIFICIAL INSEMINATION— NOT ARTIFICIAL AT ALL!

Perhaps the most exciting advance in reproductive medicine has been the development of laboratory techniques to help you get pregnant. One of the most successful is artificial insemination, a process that utilizes a simple medical procedure to place your partner's sperm (or that of a donor) inside your body at the time that you are ovulating. The actual creation of your baby then takes place *naturally* inside your fallopian tubes, the same as it would if sperm were deposited via sexual intercourse. The *only* thing artificial about insemination is the process of getting the sperm to your egg. Everything else about your pregnancy follows the natural course.

CAN ARTIFICIAL INSEMINATION HELP YOU?

Originally developed as an effective means of conceiving if your partner was not able to ejaculate and/or have an erection, today's insemination can answer the conception needs of millions of couples with a vast array of reproductive problems, including

- Marginal to low sperm counts
- Poor sperm motility
- Sperm antibodies (in you or in your mate)

278

- Seminal fluid deficiencies
- Hostile cervical mucus
- Vaginal, cervical, or uterine abnormalities

In addition, I have personally used artificial insemination to successfully treat a great number of couples with unexplained infertility, where a pregnancy cannot occur but no physiological reason can be found. Researchers theorize that minor defects in *both* partners' reproductive systems (too slight to be measured by any test) may come together to create a barrier to conception.

NOT ALL INSEMINATIONS ARE ALIKE! HOW TO TELL WHAT'S RIGHT FOR YOU

Depending on the type of physiological problem that is causing your infertility, different kinds of insemination processes are used. Each places the sperm in a different area of your reproductive tract, and each best solves a distinct set of fertility problems.

When performed with your partner's sperm, the procedure is called AIH (for Artificial Insemination Husband). If a donor sperm is used, the process is called AID (for Artificial Insemination Donor) or, most commonly, TDI (for Therapeutic Donor Insemination).

There are four basic types of insemination:

- *Vaginal insemination.* This was the first type of insemination developed. Here, sperm is placed inside your vagina and left on its own to swim up to your fallopian tubes. This method works best when your partner's sperm is good but he cannot ejaculate, or when you have unexplained infertility.
- *Intracervical insemination.* This process places sperm a little higher into your reproductive tract, at the mouth of your womb, which is located at the top of your cervix. It is often used when infertility is caused by deficiencies in your cervical mucus, by vaginal abnormalities, or when sperm has a borderline motility problem.
- *Intrauterine insemination (IUI).* One of the newest of the insemination processes, this method bypasses the vagina and cervix completely and places sperm directly into the uterus, very close to the opening of your fallopian tube. Giving sperm a strong running start, this process helps overcome infertility due to antisperm antibodies in your cervical mucus, insufficient or hostile mucus, endometriosis, irregular ovulation, low sperm count, and/or poor sperm motility.
- *Intratubal insemination.* This newest form of insemination places the sperm directly into both your fallopian tubes (if they are both healthy), as close to your egg as possible. Unlike the other forms of

insemination, this process requires that you be placed under sedation and that sperm be inseminated via a laparoscopy. Since almost all barriers in your reproductive tract are removed, fewer sperm are needed to ensure a conception. Intratubal insemination is an excellent technique for infertility due to a exceptionally low sperm count. One important requirement: you must have at least one healthy tube.

In addition to these four methods, some researchers are now experimenting with intraperitoneal insemination, placing sperm into the abdominal-pelvic cavity called the cul de sac. Preliminary results, however, show that this method is no more effective than those already in use.

PREPARING SPERM FOR INSEMINATION

When you conceive via sexual intercourse, it is your cervical mucus that transports sperm to your uterus and tubes. It is also your mucus that helps separate sperm from debris normally found in semen, such as white blood cells (which emit toxins harmful to conception), bacteria, prostaglandins (which can cause painful uterine cramping), and dead sperm.

Although vaginal and cervical inseminations do allow your partner's sperm to make contact with your cervical mucus, intrauterine insemination, by far the most successful type, does not.

To help ensure its success, a special laboratory procedure called sperm washing has been developed to simulate some of the functions of cervical mucus.

HOW SPERM WASHING IS DONE

1. The ejaculated sperm is placed in a container and left for about a half hour to liquefy at room temperature.
2. Next the sperm is mixed with a culture medium (similar to the fluid found inside your fallopian tubes) and placed into a centrifuge, a machine that spins the sperm, separating it from the seminal fluid.
3. After about ten minutes, the sperm forms a small, concentrated pellet that falls to the bottom of the container. The procedure can be repeated up to three times, depending on how much cleansing the specific sperm sample requires.
4. Unless the sperm count is exceptionally low, the sperm is now ready to be inseminated.

Although technically a vaginal or cervical insemination does not require washing (since both procedures allow for contact with cervical mucus), utilizing it in conjunction with these treatments helps raise the chances for success by allowing only the healthiest, most motile sperm to be used for the insemination.

THE SWIM-UP: MORE GOOD NEWS FOR SPERM

In cases of extremely low sperm count or exceptionally high white blood count, or when sperm morphology or motility is especially poor, a second procedure, called a swim-up, is sometimes used to further isolate the healthiest sperm.

A swim-up is performed by placing the already washed sperm pellet into a test tube containing the culture medium and then into an incubator (set at body temperature) for up to two hours. During this time, the healthiest and most motile sperm swim up to the top of the container; hence the name. Once this occurs, the sperm are gently sucked up into a hollow glass tube and loaded into a syringe, ready for insemination. The swim-up process can also be used to separate male and female sperm for the purposes of sex selection.

HEPARIN: ANOTHER WAY TO ASSIST SPERM

Another important function of cervical mucus is to initiate a process called capitization. Here, it helps trigger the release of enzymes present in the head of each sperm (the acrosome) for breaking down the hard, shell-like coating of an egg. One of the most promising new ways to duplicate these effects is the incubation of sperm in laboratory solutions of heparin (a natural body acid) and two other body chemicals just prior to insemination. Studies show this can initiate the enzymatic response necessary for conception to occur.

HOW CAFFEINE CAN HELP YOUR INSEMINATION

Recent research reports that when sperm motility is exceptionally low, meaning they simply do not swim efficiently enough to reach your egg, caffeine can help. How? Incubating washed sperm in a solution of caffeine before insemination is said to cause them to move faster. While there is no evidence to show that drinking caffeine prior to ejaculating can have the same effect, it would not be detrimental if your partner wanted to test this theory on his own.

OVULATION AND INSEMINATION: GETTING YOUR BODY READY

One of the prime ways to ensure that your insemination will be successful is to make certain that sperm is deposited at the time that you are ovulating. Using your BBT and your cervical mucus as a guide, you should begin to chart your most fertile time a month or two before your insemination is to take place. However, to be sure the timing is right, you must also use an ovulation predictor during the cycle in which you plan to be inseminated, either a kit that measures LH levels or the new Cue device (both described in Chapter Thirteen). This is the only way you and your doctor can accurately plan the day your body will be ready to receive sperm.

Depending on the method of prediction you use, your doctor can determine which signal is the one that indicates the time is right.

SUPEROVULATION: THE NEW WAY TO ENHANCE INSEMINATION

As research into reproductive endocrinology advanced, scientists began to notice that women who needed fertility drugs to make eggs actually had more successful inseminations than did those women whose ovaries and eggs were perfect. The reason, researchers theorized, was that the fertility drugs helped create healthier, stronger eggs that actually were more fertile. Thus, the concept of superovulation was applied to artificial insemination. Here, fertility drugs are given prior to insemination even if you have no egg-making problems. So successful is this treatment that most fertility clinics currently advise *all* women having insemination also to have superovulation.

THE INSEMINATION PROCESS: WHAT TO EXPECT

Within twenty-four hours of your predicted ovulation time, your insemination will take place. On the scheduled day, your partner will be asked to provide a sample of fresh sperm about two hours before the procedure. This can be done via masturbation into a sterile container provided by the lab or via sexual intercourse using a specially prepared condom. (I'll tell you how this works in a moment.)

1. As soon as the sperm has been washed, it will be aspirated into a long, thin catheter with a syringe at its end.
2. You will be asked to lie on a gyn examining table, and your feet will be placed in the stirrups. A speculum will be gently inserted into your vagina to hold it open during the procedure.
3. Next, your doctor will insert the catheter into your vagina and/or up to your cervix or your uterus. Once this is in place, he or she will slowly depress the syringe and release the sperm.
4. To help lock the insemination in place, a small plastic-covered

fertility sponge is inserted into your vagina, directly in front of your cervix. It remains in your body for about six hours, after which time you can remove it, using an attached string similar to those provided for the removal of tampons.

In an alternative method, a small plastic cap is placed over your cervix prior to the insemination. The sperm is then injected through a small opening in the cap, which snaps shut the moment the catheter is withdrawn. This prevents any chance of spillage and ensures that all the inseminated sperm remain inside your body. You remove the cap in six hours yourself.

Inseminations are completely painless and require no sedation.

NATURAL SEX:
STILL THE BEST ROUTE FOR SPERM

Until recently, most fertility programs routinely instructed your partner to obtain a sample of his sperm through masturbation, either at home or in a private room at the clinic that was equipped with magazines, soft lighting, and even adult videos. Now, however, tests conducted at the Andrology Institute in Lexington, Kentucky, show that sperm counts in semen samples obtained during *natural* intercourse were 324 percent higher than those collected in a lab. In some cases, the increase was significant enough to push men with a low sperm count into the normal range. In addition, motility was up by 16 percent, and 20 percent more normally shaped sperm appeared in men who had produced abnormal sperm in the lab.

INTERCOURSE: BETTER FOR MEN THAN MASTURBATION

Although masturbation is still utilized to supply sperm samples, especially by men making contributions to sperm banks, researchers theorize that for many men the greater degree of stimulation offered by sexual intercourse may cause more sperm to pass into the vas deferens. Sex also leads to a more intense orgasm, which, researchers report, allows more of the young, newly matured sperm lying near the epididymis to come forward and leave the body.

To utilize the benefits of intercourse for insemination, a special condom that is sterile and contains no spermicide can be worn to collect the ejaculate. The condom is brought to the lab in a sterile container and given to the embryologist, who empties it into a test tube and begins the washing process.

If sperm is collected at home, it must be kept warm during the transport. The best temperature is body temperature, and many women find that carrying the container in their bras, between their breasts, is the optimal way. If you live farther than an hour from your clinic, the embryologist can show your partner how to empty the sperm from the condom into a container filled with a special medium to preserve it for several hours.

HOW TO INCREASE THE SUCCESS OF YOUR INSEMINATION

Much the same way that lying still after natural sex can help keep sperm inside you, so, too, does minimizing movement after artificial insemination help increase its effectiveness. Although some doctors disagree, I believe that remaining on the examining table, with your buttocks raised slightly upward for about twenty minutes following your insemination will help encourage conception. In addition, I believe you should also spend at least a few hours in bed as soon as you return home. By relaxing in a nonstressed environment, it's possible you can increase your chances for a pregnancy. I have used both these techniques to encourage a successful conception in those couples who were not previously able to get pregnant via insemination before.

SHOULD YOUR PARTNER BE PRESENT DURING YOUR INSEMINATION?

If your partner wants to be a part of your insemination process, I wholeheartedly recommend that he be there every step of the way. Sharing the insemination experience can help you bond closer not only to each other, but to your baby as well. Because, however, some men find the idea of insemination very disturbing (especially if donor sperm is needed), it may be easier for him not be to present during the process. If this *is* how your partner feels, don't be alarmed; the reaction falls within the range of normal feelings. Do, however, discuss how he feels about being present well before your day of insemination. This can help you avoid any excess stress immediately prior to the procedure.

THE SECOND INSEMINATION: IS IT NECESSARY?

While the advent of advanced ovulation predictor methods have helped to time inseminations more accurately than ever, no system is infallible, and errors in timing can be made. For this reason, I strongly advocate two consecutive inseminations, forty-eight hours apart, just in case your ovulation occurred later than predicted. This is especially important if you have been stimulated via superovulation. A second insemination can raise the likelihood that sperm is deposited at the right time, thereby taking full advantage of the effects of the fertility drugs and increasing your odds for a pregnancy.

GETTING PREGNANT: HOW MUCH CAN IT COST?

Although insemination remains among the least expensive of fertility procedures being used today, it *can* still be expensive—especially since it may take several cycles before you conceive. Prices vary from one geographic location to the next and even from clinic to clinic, but these 1990 figures provide a reasonable average:

- ◆ Vaginal and/or cervical insemination: $50 to $150 per try
- ◆ Intrauterine inseminations (with sperm washing): $150 to $200 per try
- ◆ Superovulation: up to several hundred dollars per cycle, depending on the drugs used.

DOES INSURANCE COVER ARTIFICIAL INSEMINATION?

Several insurance plans cover laboratory-aided conceptions, including artificial insemination. Some, however, do not recognize any type of infertility treatment. To help cover the costs, you can sometimes schedule other gynecological treatments that *are* covered at the same time as your insemination, thus improving your chances for being reimbursed.

DONOR SPERM: INCREASING YOUR CONCEPTION ODDS

Even with new techniques like sperm washing, swim-up, and superovulation, some men simply cannot produce enough sperm, or sperm of high-enough quality, to make an insemination work. In fact, for some men sperm count can be so low that even in vitro fertilization (which requires the smallest concentration to bring about a conception) is not successful. When this is the case, you might want to consider donor sperm.

HOW DONOR SPERM IS CHOSEN

Currently more than 30,000 babies are conceived in the United States each year by donor sperm. It has become a viable alternative for many women whose partners simply can't bring about a fertilization. You can choose sperm from a sperm bank, where donors contribute anonymously, or you might want to choose the sperm of a friend or your partner's relative. In either case, sperm donors are generally chosen to match as closely as possible your partner's characteristics—primarily hair, eye and skin coloring, blood type, weight, body build, age, race, and religion. Some fertility clinics go so far as to match occupation and family background.

Your doctor and/or your fertility clinic can advise you on the selection process, as well as on the differences between fresh and frozen sperm.

SINGLE MOTHERS AND DONOR SPERM: A PREGNANCY OPTION

While the majority of women who conceive via insemination do so to overcome specific fertility problems, the procedure also opens the door for another pregnancy option: single motherhood.

As their biological clocks begin to run down before they find a suitable marriage partner, many women are now considering artificial insemination with donor sperm as a way of becoming a mother.

If your doctor refuses to inseminate you because you are single, seek another physician. Your candidacy for insemination should be based solely on your abilities to conceive, deliver, and care for a healthy baby. Do not allow any physician or clinic to judge your right to be a mother.

A FINAL WORD ABOUT INSEMINATION

No longer looked upon as a treatment for male inadequacy, like most fertility treatments, artificial insemination is viewed by today's couples as a joint effort to conceive, regardless of which partner is being treated.

Remember, too, that artificial insemination is not artificial at all. Your conception and your pregnancy will be as natural as any.

· 20 ·

THE NEW IN VITRO FERTILIZATION

How It Can Help You Conceive

In 1978 an English woman named Lucy Brown gave birth to a baby girl after having been infertile for many years. Mrs. Brown didn't realize at the time that she and Baby Louise, as the media came to call her child, would become a symbol of hope for millions of infertile couples for generations to come. What was so special about Louise? She was a test tube baby, the very first child conceived via the laboratory conception process called in vitro fertilization. Her birth was one of the medical accomplishments of the century, and it sent researchers on a journey of scientific exploration, the results of which revolutionized reproductive medicine.

HOW IN VITRO FERTILIZATION WORKS

The concept behind in vitro fertilization (IVF) is actually quite simple. It allows for fertilization to take place in an artificial environment, outside your reproductive system. It works by extracting your eggs and your partner's sperm and placing them together in a carefully controlled laboratory environment, specially developed to help foster fertilization.

If the sperm penetrates the egg and the conceptus begins to divide, indicating that fertilization has occurred, the embryo is transferred to your uterus, where it should implant and begin to grow. The remainder

287

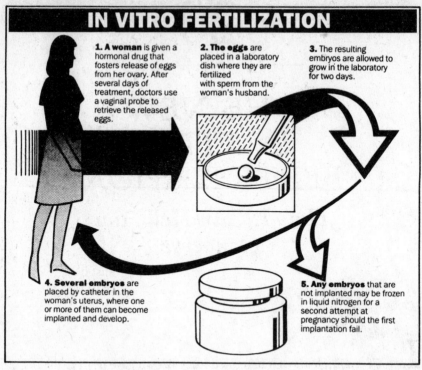

IN VITRO FERTILIZATION

1. A woman is given a hormonal drug that fosters release of eggs from her ovary. After several days of treatment, doctors use a vaginal probe to retrieve the released eggs.

2. The eggs are placed in a laboratory dish where they are fertilized with sperm from the woman's husband.

3. The resulting embryos are allowed to grow in the laboratory for two days.

4. Several embryos are placed by catheter in the woman's uterus, where one or more of them can become implanted and develop.

5. Any embryos that are not implanted may be frozen in liquid nitrogen for a second attempt at pregnancy should the first implantation fail.

Courtesy of *New York Daily News*, Rod Eyer

of your pregnancy progresses naturally, as if conception had occurred via sexual intercourse.

CAN IVF HELP YOU?

One of the chief advantages in IVF is that it allows conception to occur without the use of your fallopian tubes. Tubal damage is therefore one of the prime reasons for considering IVF. In addition, research has shown that this procedure is also highly successful in overcoming a variety of reproductive problems:

- ◆ Male factor infertility
- ◆ Unexplained infertility
- ◆ Cervical or uterine damage, especially that caused by exposure to DES
- ◆ Antisperm antibodies
- ◆ Anovulation (lack of ovulation)
- ◆ Advancing maternal age

While it may not be the first line of defense for all these problems, when other treatments (including artificial insemination) fail to help, IVF often succeeds.

PREPARING YOUR BODY FOR IVF

Because not every egg a woman ovulates is fertile, it was realized early on that the more eggs you had available for fertilization, the greater the chance for your in vitro conception to succeed. Thus the use of fertility drugs became a part of in vitro fertilization.

Currently, nearly every woman who attempts an IVF pregnancy is first treated with at least one cycle of fertility drugs, even if the eggs she produces on her own are healthy. (See the discussion of superovulation in Chapter Eighteen). Because, however, the dosages needed to make multiple eggs are generally higher than those used simply to induce the production of healthy eggs, all possible precautions must be taken to avoid hyperstimulation syndrome (again, see Chapter Eighteen). If hyperstimulation seems inevitable, all fertility medication must be immediately stopped, and your IVF cycle canceled. You will be free to try again right after the start of your next menstrual cycle.

YOUR IN VITRO EXPERIENCE: WHAT TO EXPECT

Once superovulation has occurred and your in vitro team determines that your eggs are ripe and ready for fertilization, you are ready for the egg retrieval, during which your eggs are taken from your ovary just before they would normally be ovulated. In order to retrieve your eggs your IVF team will use one of two procedures:

- *Laparoscopy.* A small incision is made into your naval, through which your doctor will insert the egg retrieval instruments.
- *Vaginal probe ultrasound.* A nonsurgical procedure, in this process your doctor attaches the egg retrieval instruments to a vaginal probe, which he then inserts into your vagina and places right next to your ovary.

In either method your doctor uses a thin, double-barreled, hollow needle inserted through your pelvic cavity to your ovary, where he or she drains the fluid from each egg follicle and deposits it in a sterile container. This is quickly passed to the embryologist, who examines the fluid and isolates the egg, being careful to set aside only those that are ripe and healthy enough for fertilization. If the fluid does contain an egg, your doctor continues to drain each of the remaining follicles until all the available eggs are retrieved. In the event that an egg becomes stuck, or agglutinated, to the side of a follicle (indicated by the lack of an egg in your follicular fluid sample), your doctor will inject a sterile fluid to release it and then retrieve it.

Although part of your in vitro procedure requires some surgery and the use of a light, general anesthesia or intravenous sedation, IVF is almost always performed on an outpatient basis.

The entire egg retrieval process takes from sixty to ninety minutes. Afterward you spend one to two hours in the recovery room, and then you are free to return home and resume most of your normal activities.

IMPORTANT NOTE

On the average, six to eight eggs are usually retrieved; of those, three to four are generally ripe enough for fertilization. However, individual egg production can vary greatly. For some women, only three to four eggs are made, with one or two ripe enough to be fertilized. For others, twelve to fifteen eggs can be retrieved, with eight or more ready for conception. Your doctor can advise you on the options concerning the amount of eggs you produce for your in vitro fertilization.

PREPARING YOUR PARTNER FOR IVF

On the day your egg retrieval is to take place, your partner will be asked to give a sperm sample. As in artificial insemination, he can do this via masturbation, at home or at the fertility clinic, or via sexual intercourse performed at home, ejaculating into a specially prepared condom (see Chapter Nineteen).

Because your partner's sperm will not be traveling through your cervical mucus as it would if you conceived via sexual intercourse, some laboratory preparation is needed before the in vitro process can succeed. As in artificial insemination, the sperm washing and swim-up procedures are normally used to ensure the highest concentration of healthy sperm. Although a successful IVF pregnancy has been achieved with sperm counts as low as one million per milliliter, the more healthy sperm concentrated in the sample, the greater the chances for conception. Finally, to maximize his sperm count, your partner should abstain from ejaculatory action for two to three days, but for no more than seven, prior to sperm collection. (Allowing more than seven days to pass without an ejaculation could cause his semen sample to be diluted with dead sperm.)

HOW AN IN VITRO CONCEPTION OCCURS

Having chosen the best and highest-quality eggs from those retrieved, the embryologist places them in an incubator, where they remain for several hours. This helps simulate the natural situation, in which your ovulated egg would spend time in your fallopian tube before reaching the area at which it makes contact with the sperm. After the incubation process, the following steps take place:

1. If sperm count is high, the eggs are individually placed in shallow glass dishes, and a portion of sperm is added to each one.
2. If sperm count is low, the eggs are placed together in one dish, and all the sperm is added to the single container.
3. After sperm and egg are combined, they are placed in an incubator, where the fertilization process should take place. It is estimated that 80 percent of all mature eggs become fertilized during the IVF procedure. If more than one sperm penetrates an egg (a situation called polyspermy), an abnormal embryo results, and that egg is not transferred to your uterus.
4. Within twenty-four hours after fertilization, your egg becomes a two-celled embryo. Within forty-eight hours, four cells result, and within sixty hours, eight cells. Your embro is ready for implantation into your uterus at any time between the two-cell and eight-cell stage. The average time is within forty-eight hours after fertilization, approximately two days after your egg retrieval.

EMBRYO TRANSFER: GIVING YOUR EGG BACK TO YOU

In the last stage of the IVF process, your doctor places your fertilized egg (the embryo) into your uterus. This is done by placing a thin plastic guide tube into your vagina and gently easing it up through your cervix and into your uterus. A thin catheter containing all the fertilized eggs is then inserted into the guide tube. A syringe attached to the outside of the catheter is gently depressed, allowing the eggs to travel through the tube and into the center of your uterus. The goal is to place the embryos so as to allow them to stick to the wall of your uterus, where, it is hoped, they will immediately implant and begin to grow.

IMPORTANT NOTE

Because not every egg that is fertilized naturally can guarantee a pregnancy, so too, not every egg that is placed into your uterus during IVF will implant and grow. This is why at least three or four eggs are usually transferred at the same time. Under certain circumstances, your doctor may even elect to deposit more. However, while your chances for conception increase with each egg that is transferred, recent studies have found that transferring more than four eggs does not significantly increase those odds. (It does increase your chances for a multiple birth.)

CONFIRMING YOUR PREGNANCY

While the excitement surrounding your IVF may indeed cause you to *feel* pregnant as soon as your embryo is transferred, it actually takes about two weeks before an implantation can be confirmed. Many of my patients have confided that this waiting period is the most difficult phase of IVF. You are not alone, however, in your anticipation. It is during this time that my in vitro team and I appreciate the fact that, for all the scientific advances, the success of our efforts is still governed by nature.

At the end of the two-week wait you will be given a pregnancy test. If the result is positive, one to two weeks later you will be given a sonogram to identify how many babies you are carrying (the average IVF birth is twins) and to confirm the fetal heartbeats.

Unless you have specific health considerations, your IVF pregnancy will not be considered high risk, unless you have a multiple pregnancy.

THE NATURAL CYCLE: A NEW ALTERNATIVE

One of the newest IVF options being explored is the all-natural cycle, using no fertility drugs. Preparation for the cycle is somewhat similar to that for fertility drugs. You are examined in the same fashion and are given sonograms every two to three days to follow the natural growth and development of your egg. You are also advised to use an ovulation predictor kit and/or blood tests for LH, to help determine when your egg is ready for retrieval. If your follicle appears to be healthy, egg aspiration, using the standard in vitro technique, is done just after your LH surge is detected. Once retrieved, your egg is fertilized in a petri dish, using the standard IVF techniques. Should conception take place, twenty-four to forty-eight hours later your embryo is transferred into your body.

This method can prove effective especially for those women unable to tolerate fertility drugs, but because only one egg is available for fertilization, chances for a pregnancy are somewhat lower than those when egg-producing medications are used.

CHOOSING YOUR IVF CLINIC

In the years since the birth of Baby Louise, IVF has proved to be extremely successful in helping millions of infertile couples get pregnant.

For this reason, there has been a great increase in the number of fertility programs offering this service.

While most of the clinics, hospitals, and private physicians performing IVF (and other new reproductive technologies) are reputable and medically qualified, like all professions, medicine has its share of charlatans. For this reason, the American Fertility Society, a long-standing international organization of reproductive endocrinologists and surgeons, has issued a set of minimum standards for all IVF programs. Before you choose a fertility program, make certain it meets these standards in regard to personnel:

◆ At least one individual has both training and experience in reproductive endocrinology, particularly in the use of fertility drugs.
◆ At least one individual has expertise in infertility surgery, including laparoscopy and the use of the vaginal probe.
◆ A director of the embryology laboratory has both training and personal experience in basic clinical embryology
◆ An ultrasonographer or obstetrician-gynecologist with specialized training and experience in reading ultra-sonograms is on staff.
◆ There is a program director, preferably a medical doctor.

Although an individual may fulfill the requirement for expertise in more than one area, I urge you to check the credentials and experience of all individuals involved in any fertility program:

◆ The *Directory of Medical Specialists,* in the reference section of most libraries, offers information on practitioners, as can the local office of your state medical society. Each local office is listed in the white pages of the phone book.
◆ Write to the American Fertility Society for reference material or information regarding clinics in your area:

  The American Fertility Society
  2140 11th Avenue South, Suite 200
  Birmingham, AL 35205-2800

◆ If possible, check with someone who has undergone an IVF; especially seek someone who was treated by the program you are considering. Networking and sharing information among infertile couples can go a long way toward achieving optimal-quality care. To find other couples in your area who are having fertility problems, contact RESOLVE, a support group/information clearing-house that offers a wealth of resources for couples considering IVF or any other fertility procedure. If you can't find a local office in your area, write to its headquarters:

RESOLVE, Inc.
5 Water Street
Arlington, MA 02174

BEFORE YOU CHOOSE A CLINIC: ANOTHER IMPORTANT CONSIDERATION

Although IVF programs are not required to offer their patients follow-up obstetrical care, the more progressive clinics throughout the world certainly do. I strongly believe that such care gives important medical and psychological continuity to your treatment. Knowing at first hand the physical circumstances that existed both during superovulation and during the egg retrieval and transfer steps can, I believe, allow your physician a better insight into how best to manage your pregnancy overall, and that could reduce your risk of miscarriage and premature labor.

For this reason I strongly suggest that you give priority consideration to those fertility programs that do offer this vital follow-up care, especially if your pregnancy will be considered high risk.

THE COSTS AND THE COVERAGE: WHAT YOU NEED TO KNOW

Depending on the comprehensiveness of your IVF program (including staff, operating facilities, and laboratory work), the cost of your conception can vary greatly, not only from clinic to clinic, but also from one geographic location to the next. In addition, the fertility drugs used for superovulation, as well as how much of these medications you need and for how long you need to take them, can influence the price as well.

On the average, an IVF procedure should cost between $5,000 and $7,000 per try (in 1990).

Does insurance cover this? Most policies and/or union plans do not cover fertility treatments, but some make an exception for IVF. Even if all the procedures are not covered, under some policies the medications used for superovulation can sometimes be reimbursed, when also used as a treatment. If it's possible to have your eggs retrieved during a procedure that is performed for other reasons, part of your IVF may be covered by insurance.

However, do not assume that your policy covers IVF, even if fertility treatments are mentioned. Ask your insurance or union representative for specifics, and get the answers and the payment guarantees in writing prior to scheduling any procedures. In addition, check with your doctor for a complete and specific breakdown of his or her charges.

WILL IVF WORK FOR YOU? HOW TO TELL BEFORE YOU TRY

One of the advancements spawned from IVF research is the Clomiphene Challenge Test (CCT), a diagnostic procedure that uses fertility drugs to help couples know if pregnancy via IVF is possible. Although not every IVF program uses CCT, those that do use the test believe it can save patients time and money by helping to predict their physiological capabilities to make eggs.

The test begins by first administering the fertility drug Clomid. Then, by measuring increases in your levels of FSH and LH (the two hormones that surge when eggs are made) at specific times in your cycle, your doctor can ascertain if you are capable of making the eggs necessary for IVF. If your hormones do not reach the recommended level, it is thought that egg production has ceased and menopause (premature or normal) has begun. In such a case, you may want to consider donor eggs (see Chapter Twenty-one).

Although generally reliable, the test is not 100 percent accurate, however, so many fertility programs question its value.

IMPROVING THE ODDS OF YOUR IVF: WHAT CAN BE DONE

Although a good portion of your IVF success is determined by the quantity and quality of your eggs and your partner's sperm, there are factors that can improve the odds for a successful conception.

MEDICATION

During the IVF procedure your doctor can preserve and protect your pregnancy by prescribing certain drug treatments:

- Ritodrine hydrochloride injection and/or ibuprofen tablets (Motrin) can cut down the uterine cramping that can sometimes cause you to expel the embryo directly after implantation. They are given just prior to your egg transfer.
- Injections of hCG and/or natural progesterone can help your uterine lining remain strong and healthy. Treatment should begin immediately after your egg transfer and continue for at least two weeks.

Natural progesterone may be continued for several more weeks if necessary.

◆ Erythromycin, 333 mg twice daily following your egg retrieval, can minimize the threat of infection.

GET BED REST

Following an IVF, you should remain in bed in the recovery room for at least two hours. Upon returning home, you should go right to bed and remain there for up to forty-eight hours. Some IVF programs advocate resuming normal activities after just two or three hours, but I believe that this extra rest, in a nonstressed environment, gives your implantation an extra measure of security. This is especially vital if you have miscarried in the past.

DO NOT SMOKE

Important new studies from Sheba Medical Center in Tel Hashomer, Israel, reveal that regular, daily cigarette smoking in almost any amount can affect the success of IVF by lowering estrogen levels, upsetting the follicular phase timing in the second half of the menstrual cycle, when your egg is fertilized and travels to your uterus). Smoking can also affect estrogen production within the egg follicle.

Nicotine in the bloodstream when your eggs are developing can affect the zona pellucida, the outside coating of your egg.

If you are contemplating IVF, give up smoking, and if possible, have your body free and clear of all traces of tobacco for at least three months prior to attempting conception.

LIMIT EXERCISE

It is vital that you limit all heavy exercise for at least the first three months of your IVF pregnancy. In addition, limit all exercise, even light workouts, for the first three weeks following your embryo transfer, extending that to eight weeks if you are prone to early miscarriage. While you don't have to lie in bed, it's important that your body is not physically overstressed or overheated during the first few important weeks of your IVF pregnancy.

PAY STRICT ATTENTION TO PRENATAL NUTRITION

All pregnant women should take prenatal vitamins and follow a balanced diet with adequate caloric intake, but it is imperative that those who conceive via IVF do so. Follow the fertility diet program in Chapter

Eleven, and take one to two prenatal vitamins a day for the duration of your pregnancy. New studies indicate that good nutrition and adequate vitamin and mineral intake prior to IVF can improve its chances for success, so follow the preparation guide in the Personal Pregnancy Planner, at the end of this book.

A FINAL WORD

There is no question that the development of IVF has helped millions of couples who would otherwise have remained infertile. Its contribution to reproductive medicine has taken our hopes and expectations beyond what we could ever have imagined. However, IVF cannot perform miracles, and more important, it doesn't always yield a conception on the first try. For many couples, two or even three IVFs are needed, so don't be discouraged if you do not get pregnant immediately.

And remember, the younger you are, the more successful your IVF is likely to be, so don't wait.

· 21 ·

THE GIFT
PROCEDURE AND
OTHER NEW
WAYS TO GET
PREGNANT . . .
PLUS HOW
TO HAVE A BABY
AFTER
MENOPAUSE

One of the aspects I found most fascinating about the technology surrounding laboratory conceptions was the possibility of combining nature and science, in such a way that we could utilize the advantages of both.

A few short years ago, Dr. Ricardo Asch, a researcher and fertility specialist working at the University of Health Science in San Antonio did just that. The result of his efforts is called the GIFT procedure. The name stands for Gamete Intra-Fallopian tube Transfer, but for the thousands of infertile couples it has already helped to conceive, it truly stands for the *gift* of life.

HOW THE GIFT PROCEDURE WORKS

In the most basic sense, getting pregnant with GIFT involves extracting mature eggs from your ovaries and then placing them together with your partner's sperm, into your fallopian tube in the precise place where fertilization is *most likely* to occur. While it draws on some of the same technology used in standard IVF, there *is* one important difference. Rather than combining egg and sperm in a laboratory, the GIFT fertilization is *all natural,* occurring inside the body, the way nature intended.

WHY CHOOSE GIFT

Many couples choose GIFT over standard in vitro fertilization simply because it is natural. However, the procedure has other advantages as well, not the least of which is its success rate, which is quite high. Recent studies show that pregnancy with GIFT is successful up to 40 percent of the time, compared to 20 percent for standard IVF, and only 14 percent for unassisted conception!

In addition, the rate of ectopic pregnancy via the GIFT procedure, less than 1 percent, is substantially lower than that for IVF, which can be as high as 10 percent, so for many women it is the safest method of assisted conception.

Why is GIFT so successful? One reason may be the fact that fertilization occurs within your body, allowing your embryo to take the natural route to implantation in just the amount of time nature intends for this journey, about five to seven days. It is during this time that your uterus makes the final preparations for a healthy implanation. Since unless it is frozen an embryo can only live outside the body for three days, for IVF your fertilized egg must be placed into your uterus two to four days sooner than it would be in the normal time frame. For many women this difference in timing is crucial to the success of their pregnancy.

CAN THE GIFT PROCEDURE WORK FOR YOU?

The success of the GIFT procedure requires that, in addition to the ability to manufacture eggs, you have at least one healthy fallopian tube. Thus it's not right for every couple. However, if the cause of your infertility is not tube related and your body can still make eggs, you are considered a good candidate for GIFT. In fact, if your doctor diagnoses any of the following fertility problems, it's highly likely that the GIFT procedure can help:

- ♦ Unexplained infertility
- ♦ Male-factor infertility

- ◆ Endometriosis
- ◆ Cervical factor infertility
- ◆ Damaged fimbria
- ◆ Lack of ovulation
- ◆ Antisperm antibodies
- ◆ Juxtaposed tube and ovary (one good tube and one good ovary on opposite sides of the body)
- ◆ Recurring ectopic pregnancy

HOW GIFT HELPS YOU GET PREGNANT

The GIFT procedure begins with the superovulation fertility drug treatments, egg monitoring, and retrieval steps used in standard IVF (see Chapter Nineteen), along with sperm-washing and swim-up technologies. At this point, however, the similarities end.

Rather than waiting in a petri dish for sperm to join them, your eggs remain out of your body for only a brief period, just long enough to aspirate all the follicles and retrieve all the eggs.

As soon as this occurs, sperm and egg are individually loaded into a syringe attached to a long, thin guide tube. Utilizing the same incision that had been used to retrieve your eggs, the tube is inserted into your pelvic cavity and through to the entrance of your fallopian tube. The syringe is gently depressed, releasing both eggs and sperm into the exact place in your tube at which they would normally have met in sexual intercourse. If enough eggs are retrieved, the same process is repeated in the opposite tube—on the average, six to eight eggs are deposited in both tubes. The catheter and the guide tube are then removed, and one small stitch closes your abdominal incision. The entire procedure takes from sixty to ninety minutes. Left on their own, the sperm and egg usually fertilize in about six to eight hours; conception is considered completely natural.

THE POST-GIFT RECOVERY

As with standard IVF, the same post-transfer precautions apply after GIFT. These include a few hours of rest in the recovery room, followed by bed rest for at least forty-eight hours at home. To increase your chances for a healthy implantation, treatment with natural progesterone injections, alone or in combination with the hormone hCG, for about two weeks, can also help.

NATURAL PREGNANCY AFTER GIFT

Perhaps one of the most exciting benefits of the GIFT procedure was something neither doctors nor researchers had anticipated: for some women, a *natural* pregnancy follows the delivery of a GIFT baby. A growing number of patients are reported to have conceived spontaneously during love-making a few months after their menstrual cycles returned.

Researchers theorize *some* of the initial obstacles to fertility may be overcome by the GIFT pregnancy: hormones are rebalanced and, through the stretching of certain organs, the ravages of scar tissue are eliminated and vital passageways reopened.

FINDING A GIFT CLINIC

Although the GIFT procedure is clearly an outstanding advance in reproductive technology, not all fertility clinics perform it. The procedure itself requires great surgical skills and places greater demands upon the embryologist. It's simply easier for the doctor to perform standard IVF, even if the GIFT procedure might be more advantageous for the patient. In some cases, standard IVF might be your best alternative, but if your tubes are in good condition, you should be offered the GIFT procedure as well. If your clinic or doctor does not give you the choice, I advise you to seek a second opinion.

THE ZIFT PROCEDURE

Just as standard IVF gave way to GIFT, so GIFT has spawned an offshoot, the ZIFT (Zygote Intra-Fallopian Transfer) procedure. Combining some of the advantages of IVF and GIFT, ZIFT fertilizes your eggs in the laboratory but then transfers the embryo to your fallopian tube, allowing it to travel to your uterus on its own and implant naturally. In addition, by fertilizing your egg before it is transferred, ZIFT has the added advantage of knowing at least from a fertilization point of view, if the procedure will be successful.

Used to treat the same fertility problems as GIFT, ZIFT also requires at least one healthy fallopian tube.

INTRAVAGINAL CULTURE: USING YOUR BODY AS AN INCUBATOR

In another new development, used in conjunction with ZIFT and IVF, your body temperature, rather than an artificial incubator, fosters egg fertilization.

After retrieval, eggs and sperm are placed inside a tiny container filled with a sterile culture medium. The small vial is then hermetically sealed and placed inside your vagina. A special vaginal diaphragm helps to hold it in place. This allows sperm and egg to fertilize in the correct temperature and atmosphere of natural body warmth.

Approximately forty-eight hours later, the container is removed from your vagina and opened. If fertilization has occurred, the embryo is transferred into your body.

DRILLING FOR BABIES

In one of the newest procedures to enable fertilization, a hole is made in your egg, allowing totally unobstructed sperm passage. Developed by embryologist Dr. Jacques Cohen and currently being researched at several leading universities, the new technique, called a partial zona dissection (PZD), is being used on eggs that are resistant to fertilization by standard in vitro procedures due to deficiencies in the enzymes in the head of the sperm. As noted earlier these enzymes normally break down the outer coating (zona pellucida) of the egg and allow passage inside. When these enzymes are deficient, drilling a hole in the egg, using either a fine needle or a chemical that dissolves the outer layer can help make it easier for sperm to pass inside. There is one drawback: more than one sperm can penetrate, creating a situation called polyspermy, in which embryos are defective and unable to develop and grow.

MICROINJECTION: NEW HOPE FOR REALLY BAD SPERM

If the number of motile sperm your partner has is severely limited, a new technique, currently under development, promises to help. Called microinjection, it places a single sperm onto the tip of an ultrafine needle and injects it into the egg's inner core. Pioneered at the Jones Institute in Norfolk, Virginia, researchers there have achieved fertilization through microinjection.

GETTING PREGNANT AFTER MENOPAUSE: NOW YOU CAN!

One of the most exciting new studies on getting pregnant shows it's now possible to extend your childbearing years almost indefinitely—even after menopause.

According to reports published in the *New England Journal of Medicine,* research conducted by Dr. Mark Sauer at the University of Southern California has shown it's now theoretically possible for a woman to have a baby at almost any age—even seventy or eighty—as long as her body is physically able to withstand gestation, labor, and delivery. The key to accomplishing this, reports Sauer, is the use of donor eggs in conjunction with in vitro fertilization.

In fact, a variety of new studies have proven that the only difference, reproductively speaking, between a pre- and postmenopausal woman is that after menopause the supply of eggs is exhausted. Barring disease or other physical trauma, your uterus remains remarkably the same throughout your lifetime. Replace those eggs, say researchers, and fertility can go on indefinitely!

USING DONOR EGGS: WHAT YOU NEED TO KNOW

The first step to a successful donor egg program is, of course, to find a suitable donor. Since unfertilized eggs are considered too fragile to withstand the freezing process (which is why a woman can't preserve her own eggs), new ones must be made fresh for each donation. Currently there are at least a half-dozen fertility centers in the United States offering a fresh egg donation program. The Cleveland Clinic in Ohio, one of the first and largest fertility clinics in the country, now has a pool of donors with a wide variety of backgrounds and physical characteristics. In much the way that sperm donors are chosen to match the characteristics of the father closely, egg donors are chosen to match the mother as much as possible.

However, because your body can have an immune system reaction causing you to reject an egg that is not your own—a problem that some researchers now believe may be more prevalent in postmenopausal women—studies show the most successful donation pregnancies are those where the egg-maker and egg-receiver are close blood relatives. The best choice for a donor would be your sister or your daughter (providing she is past puberty), followed by an aunt or a first cousin.

HOW TO CONCEIVE AFTER MENOPAUSE

Once a suitable donor is chosen, she is given fertility drugs to stimulate her egg production. Like other laboratory-aided conceptions, the more eggs that are available for fertilization, the greater the chance for pregnancy to occur. The goal in this process is for your donor to have at least four healthy eggs available for each donation.

At the same time your donor is taking fertility drugs, you will begin taking estrogen and progesterone, the hormones that rise considerably in levels as a result of a natural egg-making process, helping build a strong endometrial lining and preparing your uterus for implantation. The goal here is reach the levels that would naturally occur in your body if you were making your own eggs.

Utilizing hormone replacement therapy for you and fertility drugs for your donor, your doctor must work to synchronize, as closely as possible, your individual reproductive body chemistries.

Once your doctor determines this has occurred, the egg retrieval process can begin.

1. Using the same method as when gathering eggs for a standard in vitro fertilization (a laparoscopy or a vaginal aspiration), your donor's eggs are removed from her body.
2. Next, her eggs are inseminated in the laboratory, usually with your partner's sperm.
3. Then the egg and sperm are placed in an incubator, where it is hoped a fertilization will occur. If it does, when the resulting embryos reach the eight-cell stage—usually within forty-eight hours—they are ready to be transferred into your body.
4. Again, using the same techniques employed in standard in vitro fertilization, the embryos are transferred into your uterus, where it is hoped at least one will implant and begin to grow.

No further medications or hormones are needed beyond what may normally be required during a natural pregnancy. Your gestation, labor, and delivery proceed in much the same way they would if you had become pregnant prior to menopause. (For a more complete description of the egg retrieval–fertilization–transfer process, see Chapter Twenty.)

HOW SUCCESSFUL ARE POSTMENOPAUSAL CONCEPTIONS?

Because the procedure of postmenopausal pregnancy is still so new, statistics concerning its success are largely incomplete. However, at least in the case of Dr. Sauer's research at USC, the outcome was dramatically close to that in pregnancies in premenopausal women.

Specifically, four of the seven participants in Sauer's study (all of whom were between the ages of forty and forty-four and had undergone premature menopause) were able to conceive and deliver healthy babies. One did not conceive, one miscarried, and one had a stillborn baby—statistics that, according to Sauer, are considered on a par with those for younger women.

WHAT YOU NEED TO KNOW NOW!

As exciting as the new postmenopausal pregnancy studies have proven to be, their findings are not to be taken for granted. Don't be misled into believing that simply because postmenopausal pregnancy is possible, you can now blithely postpone childbearing with all assurance of being able to conceive for an indefinite period of time.

- While studies show postmenopausal pregnancy is now possible, it's important to realize that it is not the easiest feat to accomplish. The most important drawback is that currently the highest success rates for donor egg pregnancies occur between sisters, especially when the donor is young. So, unless you and your sister are very far apart, age-wise, chances are that by the time you are experiencing menopause, she won't be far behind. That may mean her eggs are too old for a healthy pregnancy.
- In addition, synchronizing the reproductive chemistry of any two women, even blood relatives, is not an easy task. One cycle may find your donor's eggs ready for retrieval before your uterus is ready for implantation. In the next cycle, your body may be ready but your donor's eggs may not be of a high enough quality for a healthy fertilization. As a result, the synchronization procedure can be costly and time-consuming, sometimes requiring a process called embryo freezing (explained later in this chapter) in order to work. It also requires dedication on the part of both you and your donor, as well as patience and special skills on the part of your doctor. Not all fertility specialists are qualified or even willing to work on postmenopausal pregnancies.
- Finally, it's important to note that any baby conceived via the egg donation program will have the genes of the female donor and the sperm provider, but no direct genetic link to the woman who gives birth—a factor that may present legal, emotional, and moral dilemmas for all parties concerned and throughout the child's lifetime.

I tell you these things not to dissuade you from a postmenopausal pregnancy, but only to caution you against blindly relying on this option to indefinitely postpone childbearing.

If you have already completed menopause, and especially if you are under age fifty, then donor eggs can be a wonderful way for you to fulfill your dreams of motherhood. However, I maintain that the younger you are when you try to conceive, the better your chance for success, so try to get pregnant as early in your childbearing years as is feasible for you—if possible, no later than in your midthirties. To help ensure you will be able to conceive at that time, it's a good idea to have your fertility checked at least once by your doctor (see Chapter Seven) before you reach age thirty. If a problem is found, it's important to note that, like pregnancy itself, treatments for infertility are infinitely more successful in younger women.

DONOR EGGS FOR YOUNGER WOMEN

While the technology of using donor eggs for postmenopausal women is currently garnering a lot of attention, it's also important to note that this same technology also works for younger women who, due to diseased or missing ovaries, cannot manufacture their own eggs, or because they are approaching menopause, may not have a sufficient number of quality eggs for a healthy conception. Even more successful before menopause, reliance on donor eggs may be the most effective way for some women to maximize their childbearing potential at any age.

FROZEN EMBRYOS: GREAT BABIES WHEN YOU WANT THEM

Another brand-new technology offers still another conception possibility: the chance to delay childbearing without sacrificing egg or sperm quality, which can diminish with age.

The technique is called embryo freezing. It involves retrieving your eggs and then, using your partner's sperm, having those eggs fertilized in the laboratory. The resulting embryos are then frozen and stored.

As the frozen embryos are able to last indefinitely, this process ensures you will have an embryo that is ready to be implanted into your body at any time—even after menopause. All it requires is that your uterus be prepared to accept the implantation—which can be assured by using estrogen and progesterone supplements in the cycle in which you plan to begin your pregnancy.

In addition, embryo freezing is sometimes used in donor egg pregnancies to preserve the embryo until the recipient's uterus is considered ready for implantation. This can give the fertility specialist an extra cycle or two to find the correct hormone dosage needed for the proper development of the endometrium.

One more use for embryo freezing is to preserve the extra eggs retrieved during an exceptionally fruitful in vitro fertilization or GIFT cycle. By fertilizing all the eggs at once, and then freezing some, the infertile couple can plan their family, spacing their children as they prefer, without the additional cost and trauma of an entirely new in vitro procedure each time they want to conceive.

THE EMBRYO TRANSPLANT: THE NEWEST DONOR TECHNOLOGY

Still one more conception possibility involves using your partner's sperm to artificially inseminate an egg donor. Once conception occurs and a pregnancy is verified, the embryo is gently flushed from your donor's body and placed inside your uterus. This technique is most advantageous for women who are infertile due to complete, irreversible ovarian failure, or when conception in their own bodies would risk transmitting a serious genetic disease.

The key to success with this treatment is synchronization of the menstrual cycles of both donor and recipient. It is vital that your body be ready to receive your donor's embryo five days after it has been conceived. If more than five days pass, the embryo usually cannot survive the removal process.

WHEN ANOTHER WOMAN CARRIES YOUR BABY

Finally, for those women who can conceive but cannot carry their own child (in the case of a severely damaged uterus or if you have had a partial hysterectomy), there is still one more possibility, a procedure called a *host uterus pregnancy*. This is actually the same as a donor egg pregnancy, except that this time *you* donate the egg and another woman carries your child.

The procedure involves using the in vitro process to retrieve and fertilize your egg with your partner's sperm and then transferring the resulting embryo into another woman's body for gestation and delivery. This procedure was recently performed in South Africa utilizing a mother and her daughter. The daughter was unable to carry a child due to a severe uterine defect, so the mother carried and successfully delivered her own grandchild, a healthy, robust baby girl!

As in other procedures in this chapter, the menstrual cycles of embryo donor and recipient must both be perfectly synchronized.

THE TECHNOLOGY OF CONCEPTION: A FINAL THOUGHT

When I met Gabriella and Peter, they had been trying to have a baby for over five years. A dedicated career couple, they had postponed childbearing until they were well past thirty. Gabriella had had no idea that when the time was finally right to start a family, her body would not comply. In fact, it was only after she and Peter had repeatedly tried and failed to conceive that they began to suspect something might be wrong.

A round of tests for each of them confirmed their worst fears. Gabriella was clinically infertile. The cause: endometriosis. One fallopian tube had been completely destroyed, the other somewhat damaged. In addition, Peter was found to have a marginally low sperm count, dropping Gabriella's chances for conception even further.

Their doctor at the time had advised them to give up trying and forget all notions of biological parenthood. Three other fertility specialists had echoed this advice.

"They told me I was too old to be a mother," said Gabriella, "and they chided me for having waited so long to try."

THE NEW GIFT OF HOPE

Just when they had been ready to accept their childless fate, Gabriella and Peter heard about the GIFT procedure and found a clinic to help them. Nearly two years later, however, they were still childless. Although the GIFT had produced three pregnancies, all three had ended in miscarriage.

HOW A COLLEGE REUNION LED TO PARENTHOOD

With their hopes and dreams behind them, Peter and Gabriella were once again ready accept their infertility when a college reunion turned their life around. At her twenty-year alumni celebration, Gabriella met Michelle, a friend and sorority sister she had not seen or talked to in over ten years. Within less than an hour Gabriella found herself confiding her fertility problems to her friend. As it turned out, Michelle had been plagued with similar difficulties, but she had been able to have a child. When Gabriella asked how she had succeeded, Michelle gave her my phone number. Before the day was out, Gabriella called me. With renewed hope, she scheduled an appointment.

NEW HOPE FOR THOSE WITH RECURRING MISCARRIAGE

After examining her and reviewing her records, I suggested that Gabriella try the same treatment that helped Michelle for recurring miscarriage: immunotherapy (see Chapter Fourteen). I arranged for her and Peter to start the treatment, and we followed it with another GIFT procedure. Nine months later, I helped her and Peter deliver a healthy baby girl. To them, it seemed like a miracle. Little did they know that another miracle was just around the bend.

THE SURPRISE OF A LIFETIME!

Within five months of the birth of their daughter, Alexandra, Gabriella came to my office feeling a little out of sorts. She was, she said, feeling very emotional and highly fatigued. She was concerned, too, about having had only one menstrual period since giving birth. Gabriella was sure she was starting menopause.

From the moment I saw her, I had a feeling about what was wrong. Two days later, test results confirmed my feelings. Gabriella was pregnant, only this time the conception had taken place spontaneously and quite naturally, with *no* outside assistance of any kind. She and Peter delivered their second child, a healthy, robust boy they named Armand.

Imagine! From hopelessly infertile to the mother of two—in less than two years.

YOU CAN HAVE A BABY!

If I could choose any era in which to practice as a gynecologist-obstetrician, I would unequivocally choose the present because of couples like Peter and Gabriella, happy, new parents who just a few short years ago would have been considered hopelessly infertile. Thanks to advances in reproductive science, most couples who want to have children can have them. Being able to offer the joy of natural parenthood to so many has brought new meaning to my career. So, don't give up. Don't accept your infertility. Today, more than ever, a miracle baby can be yours!

IV

◆

YOUR PERSONAL PREGNANCY PLANNER

• 22 •

A SIX-MONTH
GUIDE TO A SAFE
AND HEALTHY
CONCEPTION

In addition to following whatever suggestions your doctor makes during your preconception exam, *you* can also help get your body ready for a safe and healthy pregnancy. Whether you are just beginning to plan your pregnancy and believe you will be conceiving naturally or you have failed to get pregnant and have decided on a laboratory-aided conception, my personal pregnancy planner can help you have a faster, easier, and, most important, healthier conception *when you want to.*

HOW THE PERSONAL PREGNANCY
PLANNER WORKS

Based on the latest medical research and many hours of conversation with my patients, I have developed this six-month program to eliminate a good number of the obstacles to conception. Depending on your circumstances, this program could take you more or less than six months to complete. However, for most of my patients, that time period is adequate for laying the foundation for a healthy pregnancy.

To illustrate how the Personal Pregnancy Planner works, I've chosen July as the target date for conception. The months in which *you* take these steps will depend, of course, on the conception target date that you and your partner select. To chart the correct months in your own pregnancy timetable, simply count back six months prior to your target date (exclude your conception month from that count).

313

COUNTDOWN CALENDAR OF EVENTS
(TARGET DATE FOR CONCEPTION: JULY)

JANUARY: PRECONCEPTION MONTH SIX

GOAL: To be free of as many potentially toxic substances as possible by the time you conceive.

STRATEGY: Begin the elimination of alcohol, tobacco, caffeine, recreational drugs, diet pills, sugar, artificial sweeteners, diet sodas.

HELPLINES: If you are seriously addicted to any of these substances, especially if you are dependent on one or more, consider getting professional help in overcoming your habit before finalizing your target conception date.

FEBRUARY: PRECONCEPTION MONTH FIVE

GOAL: To achieve the best weight for a healthy conception.

STRATEGY: Use the chart in Chapter Nine to establish your ideal preconception weight, and come as close to that as possible within the next three months.

If you need to lose weight, avoid crash diets, diet pills, any form of fasting or starvation and liquid diets.

If you need to gain weight, add calories in the form of complex carbohydrates and protein, rather than fats. Also avoid commercial weight-gain products.

HELPLINES: Because dieting often causes tricky shifts in hormonal activity, some of which can affect your fertility, preconception weight loss or gain must be sensible and slow. In addition, because even these slow changes in body fat can have some effect on reproductive biochemicals, your system needs time to stabilize after any significant weight changes before you attempt conception.

Unless drastic losses or gains are required, you should be able to achieve your goals within three months and then use the eight to ten weeks that follow to stabilize your system before conceiving.

MARCH: PRECONCEPTION MONTH FOUR

GOAL: To overcome nutritional deficiencies that could affect your fertility and/or the health of your baby.

STRATEGY: Follow the Fertility Diet Program featured in Chapter Eleven, and remember to take one to two prenatal vitamins daily starting now. In addition, add supplements of vitamin C, folic acid, and zinc if you smoke, drink alcohol, or take birth control pills. Also important:

- Avoid junk food, preservatives, processed foods, sugar, artificial sweeteners, caffeine.
- Eat fresh fruits and vegetables, nondairy sources of calcium, and fiber, and drink lots of water!

APRIL: PRECONCEPTION MONTH THREE

GOAL: To avoid fertility- or pregnancy-related complications that arise from medication and/or birth control pills.

STRATEGY:

- Discontinue taking birth control pills, and substitute a barrier form of contraception for a period of at least three months.
- Limit the use of unnecessary medication, both prescription and over-the-counter drugs, including cold remedies, pain relievers, sinus medications, cough medicines, diet pills, diuretics, tranquilizers, and antibiotics.

HELPLINES: Should your doctor prescribe any medications during the preconception period, make certain that he or she is aware of your target date, and ask whether the drugs in question could have adverse reproductive effects. If they could, wait at least thirty (and better, sixty) days after discontinuing medication before attempting conception.

Once you stop taking them, all traces of birth control pills are normally out of your body in several weeks; however, each woman's metabolism is unique, so residues can sometimes remain longer than the average.

The risk of birth defects is slightly higher for babies accidentally conceived while birth control pills are being used, so it's wise to remain pill-free for at least three months prior to conception.

MAY: PRECONCEPTION MONTH TWO

GOALS:

- To ensure that all previously diagnosed medical problems are under control.

- To ensure that no fertility-robbing conditions have developed since your last exam.
- To establish your ovulation pattern.

STRATEGY:

- See your doctor for a follow-up preconception counseling exam; this is extremely important if you are currently using an IUD for birth control.
- Begin establishing your BBT chart and your cervical mucus patterns, as described in Chapter Thirteen.

HELPLINES: Although your first prepregnancy checkup should have included all the tests and diagnostic procedures needed prior to pregnancy, this second visit, six to eight weeks before your target conception date, is important as well, especially if you have been using birth control pills or if you use an IUD. Your second exam should include the following steps:

1. A review of your records and follow-up inspection for previously diagnosed problems
2. Removal of the IUD, followed by a repeat test for chlamydia and a prescription of 250 mg of tetracycline antibiotic taken four times a day for seven days, which will help stop the spread of any infection that can follow IUD removal.
3. A pelvic exam to ensure that no fertility-related abnormalities have developed since your previous checkup, including fibroid tumors, ovarian cysts, endometrial lesions, or adhesions.

JUNE: PRECONCEPTION MONTH ONE

GOAL: To achieve maximum fertility potential.

STRATEGY:

- Limit alcohol consumption.
- Avoid all recreational drugs.
- Stop any dieting.
- Keep exercise to a minimum.
- Avoid stress.
- Avoid caffeine.

HELPLINES: Although it's vital that you clear your body of all potentially toxic substances *before* attempting conception, it's also important that changes in your life be gradual and not abrupt. Any sharp decline in activity or sudden alteration in body chemistry (even for the better) can throw your reproductive system into a frenzy and actually keep you from conceiving, sometimes for a year or even longer. For best results, cut down negative factors *gradually,* giving your body time to adjust before you try to conceive.

JULY: YOUR TARGET CONCEPTION MONTH

If you have followed the six-month prepregnancy program *and* all the advice of your physician, you should be ready for the fast, easy conception of a healthy baby. However, it's important to keep your conception schedule flexible. Even the healthiest couples don't always conceive when they want to, so remain relaxed and confident even if a pregnancy does not occur right away.

Remember:

- It can take up to a year to get pregnant, even if you and your partner are in perfect health.
- The success rate for pregnancy in healthy, normal couples is only 14 percent, with only three possible pregnancies for every twenty-five acts of intercourse during your most fertile time.

THE MAIN THING TO REMEMBER: One of the best ways to get pregnant is to be relaxed and feel good about yourself and about the idea of becoming a parent. Use the Personal Pregnancy Planner as a guide, but don't get bogged down with routines and schedules, especially in lovemaking. Keep your sex life spontaneous and fun!

THE FORTY-EIGHT-HOUR CONCEPTION BOOST: SUREFIRE WAYS TO INCREASE YOUR FERTILITY RIGHT BEFORE YOU CONCEIVE!

THINGS YOU SHOULD AVOID

- Pantyhose
- Artificial sweeteners
- Excessive sugar
- Cola beverages, especially diet sodas
- Coffee, tea, chocolate
- Hot tubs, hot showers, saunas, steam rooms
- Heating pads and electric blankets
- Exercise
- Stress

THINGS YOUR PARTNER SHOULD AVOID

- Sex, including masturbation
- Tight underwear
- Tight pants
- Hot tubs, hot showers, saunas, steam rooms
- Heating pads and electric blankets
- Heavy physical activity

WHAT YOU AND YOUR PARTNER SHOULD DO

- Avoid stress.
- Increase vitamin C by 500 mg twice daily.
- Increase vitamin B complex by 50 mg three times daily, B_6 by 100 mg daily.
- Get at least eight hours of sleep a night for two nights.
- Avoid any use of alcohol or drugs.
- Think about making love, not about making babies.

HOW POSITIVE EMOTIONS CAN HELP YOU CONCEIVE: NINE SUGGESTIONS FOR A HAPPY, HEALTHY PREGNANCY

One of the newest theories, presented at a recent international fertility conference in Helsinki, Finland, concerns the benefits of positive emotions for couples trying to conceive. Much as negative emotions can *inhibit* reproduction, positive thoughts and strong images of a happy, healthy pregnancy can *increase* your ability to get pregnant. I have found positive emotions to play a profound role in overcoming many barriers to good health, especially those that block fertility, as I have seen emotions be a major deciding factor in cases of unexplained infertility.

For this reason, I strongly advise that you look forward not only to *getting* pregnant, but to *being* pregnant. To achieve a positive state of mind, try the following suggestions in the months and weeks prior to your conception target date:

1. *Enjoy your pregnancy preparations.* The time you spend getting ready to get pregnant should not be viewed as hard work, even though you may be working very hard indeed to achieve your goals. Feel positive about what you're doing and know in your heart that each step you take is bringing you that much closer to giving birth to a healthy, beautiful baby.
2. *Feel positive about making changes.* Don't dwell on negative feelings of deprivation even if you have to give up lifelong habits like cigarettes or caffeine.

3. *Relax about your prepregnancy goals.* Don't get uptight if you aren't accomplishing your goals on schedule. Pregnancy preparation is not a race or a competition, just a method of helping you conceive a healthy child. It is something you can enjoy, and at your own pace.
4. *Become dedicated to having a baby.* Don't let the desire to have a baby run your life, but do feel your commitment deep inside you, and feel good about that commitment.
5. *Eliminate stress—as much as possible.* Don't worry about your pregnancy or your ability to conceive. Believe you are doing everything right. Feel relaxed about not only *getting* pregnant, but *being* pregnant.
6. *Think about the joys of parenthood.* Concentrate on your happiness about being a parent, and believe that your child will be happy, healthy, and strong.
7. *Feel your fertility.* Several times during the day, close your eyes for a few moments and feel the power within you to create a wonderful, beautiful baby. Feel your body working *for* you, and begin to imagine a child growing inside you.
8. *Think about being in love, not just about making babies.* Never forget the role of love as well as love making in conception. Focus on the love that you and your partner share. Feel not only the unification of your bodies, but the coming together of your hearts and your spirit in the form of a brand-new life.
9. *Believe in yourself.* If you embrace only one positive thought in the months prior to getting pregnant, let it be a belief in yourself and your ability to conceive and deliver a healthy baby.

Never forget the power that you can have over your body and your pregnancy when you become a partner in your own health care. Believe that you can make a difference—and that what you do, say, think, and feel *are* as important as a doctor's diagnosis. Understand that sometimes what you feel in your heart can correctly contradict the most learned medical opinion.

Most of all, believe in what you're doing and your ability to make positive things happen in your life, including pregnancy. You deserve the joy of parenthood. It can and will be yours.

RESOURCES

ORGANIZATIONS

To learn more about protecting your fertility and expanding your childbearing options, the following nine organizations can help.

American College of Obstetricians and Gynecologists
409 12th Street SW
Washington, DC 20024-2188
(202) 638-5577

American Fertility Society
2140 Eleventh Avenue South
Suite 200
Birmingham, AL 35205-2800
(205) 933-8494
Free list of IVF clinics, $1 guide (in 1990) to selecting the right one

American Society of Andrology
309 West Clark Street
Champaigne, IL 61820
(217) 356-3182

American Urological Association Inc.
1120 North Charles Street
Baltimore, MD 21201
(301) 727-1100

Endometriosis Association
8585 North 76th Place
Milwaukee, WI 53223
1-800-992-3636 (in United States)
1-800-426-2363 (in Canada)

HERS (Hysterectomy Education Resources and Services)
501 Woodbrook Lane
Philadelphia, PA 19119
(215) 247-6232

National Network to Prevent Birth Defects
Box 15309 S.E. Station
Washington, DC 20003
(202) 543-5450

Nine to Five, National Organization of Working Women
614 Superior Avenue NW
Cleveland, OH 44113
(216) 566-9308

RESOLVE
5 Water Street
Arlington, MA 02174
1-800-662-1016
Self-help for infertile couples, physician referrals, IVF information, etc.

EXPERTS IN THE FIELD OF REPRODUCTIVE MEDICINE

The following is a partial listing of the private physicians, hospital and university programs offering treatment, and/or research in all areas of reproductive medicine.

Albert Einstein College of Medicine
Fertility and Hormone Center
20 Beacon Hill Drive
Dobbs Ferry, NY 10522
(914) 693-8820

Richard D. Amelar, M.D.
137 E. 36th Street
New York, NY 10016
(212) 532-0635
Specialty: male reproductive problems.

Ricardo H. Asch, M.D.
12555 Garden Grove Boulevard
Suite 203
Garden Grove, CA 92668
(714) 638-1500

Baylor College of Medicine
Department of Obstetrics and Gynecology
#1 Baylor Medical Plaza
Houston, TX 77054
(713) 798-7500

Brigham and Women's Hospital
IVF Program
75 Francis Street
Boston, MA 02115

Cleveland Clinic Foundation
IVF Program
9500 Euclid Avenue
Cleveland, OH 44106

Columbia Presbyterian Medical Center
Presbyterian Hospital IVF Program
622 West 168th Street, PH 16
New York, NY 10032

Professor Ian Craft
London Fertility Center
Cozen's House
112A Harley Street
London, W1N1AF, England
011-071-224-0707

Richard P. Dickey, M.D., Ph.D.
Fertility Institute of New Orleans
6020 Bullard Avenue
New Orleans, LA 70128
(504) 246-8971

Duke University Medical Center
Department of Obstetrics and Gynecology
Box 3527
Durham, NC 27404

Genetics and IVF Institute
Fairfax Hospital
3020 Javier Road
Fairfax, VA 22031

Hospital of the University of Pennsylvania
Department of Obstetrics and Gynecology
3400 Spruce Street
Suite 106
Philadelphia, PA 19104

IVF Australia at United Hospital
406 Boston Road
Port Chester, NY 10573

The Johns Hopkins Hospital
Division of Reproductive Endocrinology
600 North Wolfe Street
Baltimore, MD 21205

Jones Institute for Reproductive Medicine
Eastern Virginia Medical School
Hofheimer Hall, 6th Floor
825 Fairfax Avenue
Norfolk, VA 23507

Richard Mars, M.D.
Cedars–Sinai Hospital
Center for Reproductive Medicine
444 South San Vincente Boulevard, 11th floor
Los Angeles, CA 90048

Michael Reese Hospital and Medical Center
IVF-ET Program
31st Street at Lake Shore Drive
Chicago, IL 60616

Mount Sinai Medical Center
IVF Program
1212 Fifth Avenue
Box 1175
New York, NY 10029

Northwestern Memorial Hospital
IVF Program
Prentice Womens Hospital
333 East Superior Street
Suite 454
Chicago, IL 60611

J. Victor Reyniak, M.D.
1107 Fifth Avenue
New York, NY 10128
(212) 410-4080

Zev Rosenwaks, M.D.
New York Hospital–Cornell Medical Center
Obstetrics and Gynecology Department
530 East 70th Street
Room M 036
New York, NY 10021
(212) 472-5003

Jonathan Scher, M.D.
1126 Park Ave.
New York, NY 10021
(212) 427-7400
Miscarriage specialist

Geoffrey Sher, M.D.
Pacific Fertility Center
2100 Webster Street
Suite 220
San Francisco, CA 94115
(415) 923-3344
      or
Northern Nevada Fertility Institute
350 West Sixth Street
Suite 3AB
Reno, NV 89503

John J. Stangel, M.D.
70 Maple Avenue
Rye, NY 10580
(914) 967-6800

UMDNJ, New Jersey Medical School, Newark
Center for Reproductive Medicine F342
150 Bergen Street
Newark, NJ 07103

University of California at Irvine Memorial Hospital
2880 Atlantic Avenue
Suite 220
Long Beach, CA 90806

University of Texas Health Science Center
Department of Reproductive Science
6431 Fannin
Suite 3204
Houston, TX 77030

University of Texas—SW Medical School
Division of Reproductive Endocrinology
Department of Obstetrics and Gynecology
Dallas, TX 07232

University of Wisconsin
Madison Infertility Clinic
600 Highland Avenue
H4/630 CSC
Madison, WI 53792

Vanderbilt University
Center for Fertility and Reproductive Research
IVF Program
D-3200 Medical Center North
Nashville, TN 37232

Women's Health Center
University of Minnesota VIP Program
Department of Obstetrics and Gynecology
Box 395 Mayo Memorial Building
420 Delaware Street SE
Minneapolis, MN 55455

Yale University Medical School
Department of Obstetrics and Gynecology, IVF Program
333 Cedar Street
New Haven, CT 06510

INDEX

About the Authors

NIELS H. LAUERSEN, M.D., Ph.D. is a fertility specialist and the author of more than a hundred scientific papers as well as seven best-selling woman's health care books. He is a founding member of the New York Society for Reproductive Medicine, a fellow of the American Fertility Society, and a member of the American Board of Obstertricians and Gynecologists. He is also the medical director of The New York Medical Service for Reproductive Medicine, a private fertility clinic in New York City.

COLETTE BOUCHÉZ is an investigative medical reporter who writes a weekly medical column for *The New York Daily News*. Ms. Bouchéz is a member of the American Medical Writers Association and frequently lectures on women's health care issues. She lives in New York City.